Now What?

An Insider's Guide to Addiction and Recovery

William Cope Moyers

Hazelden®

Hazelden
Center City, Minnesota 55012
hazelden.org

Printed in the United States of America

Library of Congress Cataloging-in-Publication Data

Moyers, William Cope.
Now what? : an insider's guide to addiction and recovery / William Cope Moyers.
p. cm.
ISBN 978-1-61649-419-3 (softcover) — ISBN 978-1-61649-452-0 (e-book)
1. Addicts—Rehabilitation. 2. Substance abuse—Treatment. I. Title.
HV4998.M693 2012
616.86—dc23
2012027417

Editor's note
The names, details, and circumstances may have been changed to protect the privacy of those mentioned in this publication.

This publication is not intended as a substitute for the advice of health care professionals.

Alcoholics Anonymous, AA, and the Big Book are registered trademarks of Alcoholics Anonymous World Services, Inc.

16 15 14 13 12 1 2 3 4 5 6

Cover design by David Spohn
Interior design and typesetting by Madeline Berglund

To people ready to change,
and those ready to help them

CONTENTS

ACKNOWLEDGMENTS

In a book like this, it is impossible to give credit to each individual who has influenced me and what I've written. The *Now what?* asked by so many comes my way via letters, e-mails, and phone calls from people I have never met and never will. Their personal experiences are the essence of my perspective, as is the professional knowledge of researchers, scientists, and counselors who've been at it a lot longer than I have. Then there's the wisdom that I've liberally borrowed from my "fellow travelers" in long-term recovery and from those who are counting days since their last buzz. There is very little, if any, of my own original thought here. To all of these people goes the credit.

But I owe special thanks to my colleagues at Hazelden, especially Sid Farrar, the editor who pushed me to do this book. Publisher Nick Motu (who wears many hats) supported it from start to finish. And then there's Mark Mishek, the CEO. He is uniquely adroit at balancing the mission and the margin of a burgeoning organization that employs people like me and endorses books like this one. That I get to work at Hazelden is a gift beyond anything I was promised when I was a patient there so long ago.

Without Pat Samples this book would just be a good idea whose time hadn't come. Thanks, Pat, for pulling me out of my own head and getting my ideas framed into a coherent structure on a computer screen and, ultimately, on these pages. Every writer deserves an editorial consultant like you.

On her own time, Kat Joachim, my assistant at Hazelden, categorized my materials—letters, e-mails, and columns—into themes for my research.

Dr. Omar Manejwala knows addiction medicine inside and out. He made himself available at every moment I had a question demanding an immediate answer.

My agent, Amy Williams, knows the art of the deal and the deal in the art of my recovery advocacy, which is so vital to my professional duties and personal passion. She made sure this book satisfies both.

In 2007, Rick Newcombe at Creators Syndicate prompted me to start writing a weekly column on addiction-related issues. With his support, I'm still doing it. These hundreds of columns continue to elicit readers' questions, and many of my answers to them ended up in this book.

Thank you, Brad Martin, for allowing me to write a key chapter or two at your nurturing home at Blackberry Farm in Tennessee. I should write more books more often there.

When I doubted my staying power to move through these chapters while keeping pace with the rest of my life, Nell Hurley stuck with me and cheered me on. She still does, whether I waver or not.

My parents have been with me every step of the way and still are. I'm a fortunate son.

Thomas, Nancy, and Henry, my three children, encourage their father to be a writer too, even when it happens at home at my desk at night and on weekends. Their support is priceless. I relish their unrelenting love. I'm a blessed father.

FOREWORD

Our son says he dedicated his first book, *Broken,* to his parents because we were with him "every step of the way."

Ha!

He was too drunk and drugged to see how many times his father, in particular, stumbled. It seemed to me that every other time I put my foot down, I stumbled.

Or fell into quicksand.

I was ignorant, and even in the light, ignorance trips you up. When a giant hole opened in our lives, and he tumbled headfirst toward the bottom, we were sucked down with him. And in the darkness, ignorance almost devoured me.

What did I know about addiction? I was in my fifties and had never indulged in a joint (I'm seventy-eight now and still the oldest square on the block).

And alcoholism? I knew my grandfather died a drunk. And I had an uncle whose drinking made him such a malcontent that after he struck my father in a woozy state of belligerence, I had him arrested. But every town in East Texas had a handful like him, and the good folk passing just shook their heads and said, "What a shame."

I thought of alcoholism as too many drinks, not as a disease. I thought it was for other people's kin.

Our son, an alcoholic and addict? Disappearing at age thirty—without a word to his wife, not even a note to his parents, a tip-off to his brother and sister, a call to his boss? It couldn't be.

But it was. And we fell through the gates of hell and were swallowed up.

I do not exaggerate. That's how I remember it all these years later: swallowed up in frantic searches, detox, primary care, halfway houses, reassurances, consultations, lies, relapses, tears, sleepless nights, spasms of anger, pangs of fear, hallucinations, dreams of a lifeless body sprawled on a crack house floor. I hated what he was doing to himself. Hated what he was doing to us. Once—no, twice, or was it three times?—I screamed aloud, alone in my car, "E-n-o-u-g-h! I'm giving up!"

But *he* didn't give up—how could I? He hung in there, clawed his way back from the bottom, prayed, confessed, read, listened, learned, plumbed the depths of his soul, found fresh pools of courage, gained discipline, garnered wisdom, and grounded his recovery in sharing his story, unashamedly, with others.

And one day he was back. A leader in the field. An inspiration to others. A father to his children. A stalwart in his community. And the embodiment of a journey with no end and no destination and measured one day at a time.

Yes, I stumbled and fell and, at times on my knees, I was uncertain I could get up. But in the midst of his own struggle, he reached out for help—to his wife, friends, fellow travelers on the road back, kindred spirits, and yes, to his parents—and recovery became more than a solo flight; it became a mutual affair.

You will find the reasons in this book. You will see what can be learned from other parents experiencing a hell of their own and seeking the road back. I will never forget the first day at the family program when he was in treatment and a family of five from a Southern city—the father a successful banker and leader in the community—trooped in like bedraggled creatures who had been caught in a rainstorm: their oldest child had just arrived in treatment, too, and they were just as bewildered as I was. I never felt alone after that and slowly came to see addiction as a disease from which no family is immune.

William Cope has written this book for you—for those of you fighting back against a cunning disease, but he has also written it for those who love you and won't give up. It is their journey too. And like these pages, it is marked with hope.

— *Bill Moyers*

Caught completely off guard when my son crashed in 1989, I floundered in misery and anxiety.

In spite of the reality of the terrible August day when I, with the help of a friend, tracked him down in a Harlem apartment and confronted him in that doorway, I found it impossible to believe that my thirty-year-old son was a drug addict. He was one of the "golden boys" of our community, a college graduate who had a lovely wife and a great job. How could he be one of "them," the down-and-out and degraded people I saw daily on the streets of New York?

Frightened almost to death, knowing that he was in a life-or-death situation, I still found it difficult to face any friend or professional associate to get the urgent information we so desperately needed. What on earth were we to do to help him?

After a few days, my husband and I began to realize that we must have help, and we reached out and began the long journey toward recovery. Very soon I realized that I could not do this alone and fortunately was guided toward a Twelve Step group in which I found immediate relief from the terrible anxiety that was affecting me day and night.

Here was support from others who also had beloved family, friends, or colleagues suffering the pain and struggle of addiction. Only these people could possibly know what I was experiencing, and I learned from them the three C's: I did not *cause* my son's addiction, I could not *control* it, and I could not *cure* it. We signed up for the family program at Hazelden and became immersed in learning the facts about addiction—and also about the possibilities of recovery.

But I had so much more to learn. Although my counselor at Hazelden warned me that relapse following treatment was not uncommon and that I should be prepared for anything in the roller coaster of his recovery journey and mine, I convinced myself that such statistics surely did not apply to my son. Within months I had to confront the fact that relapse was a reality, an ever-present threat.

And with that growing understanding of the nature of addiction as a chronic illness, I began a deeper kind of recovery for myself. I introduced myself at Twelve Step meetings as "I'm Judith, and I am a fixer." When I admitted to myself that I had been a fixer all my life and that I had to recover from that, I began a new journey. So many of my lifelong commitments to positions of leadership and responsibility had paid off in both my professional and my personal life. My challenge now was to step back, to practice knowing the difference between fixing things and fixing people. It isn't easy.

As a start, I had to "let go" of my son's recovery. I never let go of my deep and abiding love for him, but I needed to be sure boundaries were understood and that my own health and well-being must be my first responsibility. Today I can say that I accept the challenge of "one day at a time" living. And I am so grateful that there is always hope and help.

— *Judith Moyers*

INTRODUCTION

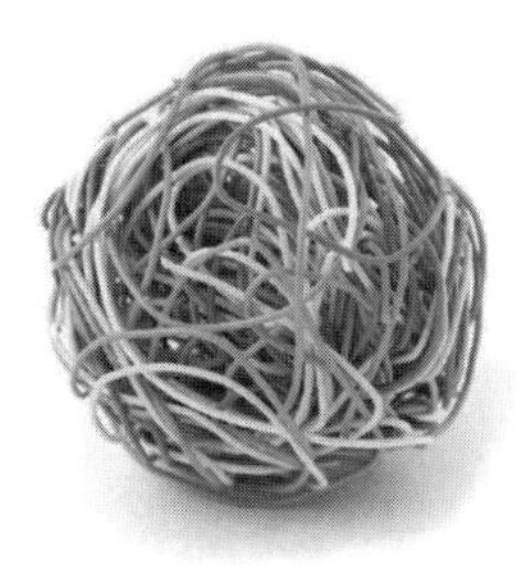

"Help, My Son Is Dying!"

Since you've picked up this book, you probably already know the helplessness, desperation, and fear of someone doing too much drinking or drugging. You know someone deeply hurt from this experience—someone you love, someone who loves you, a member of your family, a friend, co-worker, neighbor, or an elder where you worship. Perhaps that someone is you. It's me too.

I am not a doctor or a psychologist or a researcher. I am not a therapist or a clinical expert. But every day people reach out to me for advice about an incurable illness that leads to shame, confusion, and isolation. Why? Because I have never been shy about sharing my story of a long-term love affair with alcohol and other drugs—a selfish relationship. Initially that relationship was all about me, but in the end, it became only about the substances that drove me insane and almost killed me, more than once. My story is about what happens when substances hijack the vulnerable brain and steal the restless soul. It's a story I know you understand something about or you wouldn't be reading this book. It is your story or the story of somebody you know who needs help right now. There are millions of people just like us, millions of families like ours. You are not alone.

I share my story because I can; I survived the insidious spiral downward. I survived despite several devastating relapses, each worse than the one before. Not everyone has to hit bottom or go to treatment more than once. But I did. It took four treatments over five years before I finally learned to listen to what others told me and to follow their leads. So mine is not only a story of my struggle to survive, but also one of hope and rebirth. I am now in long-term recovery from alcoholism and drug dependence. My last relapse was in a crack house in Atlanta on October 12, 1994. Since then, I have been clean and sober through some very difficult years, one day at a time.

The first time I revealed my recovery from alcoholism to the public was as the featured speaker at a Rotary Club luncheon in my hometown of St. Paul, Minnesota, in 1997, and then only by accident. I was supposed to talk about drug policy and the impact of addiction in communities, but my fact-filled, antiseptic speech fell on deaf ears. Midway through, I abandoned it, instead telling my personal story. That day the audience was shocked that the son of prominent and successful parents, a community leader in my own right, a homeowner, a taxpayer, a father, and (except for a speeding ticket or two) a law-abiding citizen was also an alcoholic and addict. In their eyes I certainly didn't look like one. Yet as the people in the audience that day learned, and as I want you readers to know as well, addiction does not discriminate. Thus began my vocation to carry the message about addiction, its treatment, and how people can recover from it to everyone willing to listen to my story. I do this not just in my role at Hazelden, where I work to change public attitudes and public policy, but from a sense of personal vocation that came from the belief deep within me that giving voice to my story was necessary for my own recovery. Other people need help to overcome the same illness I had, and I am in a unique position to provide such help. That need was confirmed after I spoke at that Rotary meeting, when people began to seek me out, looking for advice for people they knew, or for themselves.

They wrote letters, sent e-mails, or called me in the middle of the night. They stopped me on the street. Sometimes strangers knocked on my front door unannounced. I believe that what drew them to contact me was that my experiences were a lot like theirs; the common denominator of our stories is the crisis of addiction and the urgency to overcome it. And since I wasn't famous or didn't have an unlisted phone number or live within a gated community, what I knew was accessible to them directly through me. It helped, too, that the institution I represented has been treating people like me since 1949.

I was primed but always surprised when, in ones or twos, people from my community reached out to me each week. I recognized that here was my opportunity to reinvest some of what my family and I had been freely given years before: practical information from real people whose own experiences bridged the span between the confusion of a life-threatening problem and the clarity of a solution. For me the added bonus was—and still is—that in giving away information and help, I get back as much as or more than the people who seek me out receive.

Yet I was totally unprepared for what happened in 1998, when my parents and I appeared on Oprah Winfrey's show to promote the *Moyers on Addiction: Close to Home* documentary television series on PBS. When she asked me, "William, what should people do when they need to get help?" I offered Hazelden's 24-hour help line phone number (now 1-800-257-7810). I didn't realize how many desperate people were watching. In the first hour after *The Oprah Winfrey Show* aired that day, Hazelden received 2,000 phone calls, which temporarily shut down the resource center that is the heart and soul of Hazelden's connection to the outside world. I will never forget hearing one of those calls forwarded to me; it was from a man in Pittsburgh who said, "Mr. Moyers, I am sitting in my living room with a loaded gun in my mouth, and if you don't help me stop drinking right now, I am going to kill myself."

From standing at the podium of a small city's Rotary Club to a year later being in the national spotlight of *Oprah, Larry King Live,* National Public Radio, and the *New York Times,* I realized my story had become a beacon for people lost in the darkness of their illness. My memoir, *Broken: My Story of Addiction and Redemption,* published eight years later, became a way for me to extend even further the light of recovery to others like me and to families like mine.

One of them is Marcy S., from Ohio. Her letter became a catalyst for this book:

> Dear Mr. Moyers,
> **Help, my son is dying.** I read your book that says to hate this disease, not the person. But so help me God, I hate him more than I love him right now. . . .

She went on to tell me the story of her son, Scott, and her struggle with his addiction. She signed off with this:

> . . . I am begging you, if there is any way my son can be helped, please help me to find it. Please help Scott to save himself, Mr. Moyers. You are my last hope.

This book, *Now What?,* is intended as a straightforward guide based on my insights in helping people like Marcy and Scott and the countless others who turn to me as their "last hope." It's not a retelling of my story, although my experiences illustrate certain points. I draw a lot from other resources and people who know more than I do, including experts in the science of addiction, data about the effectiveness of treatment, and the well-tested pathways of recovery that have worked for millions of people through the years.

Some information—people's common questions and stories—also comes from my column, *Beyond Addiction,* syndicated by Creators. Rick Newcombe, the president and CEO, gave me the opportunity to write a weekly column for his website beginning in 2007.

Most of all, I hope that in these pages you'll find practical guidance with straightforward answers to what are often perplexing questions. Those questions and responses come from the experiences of insiders who were once where you are right now.

We know that addiction is a cunning and baffling illness that isn't easy to overcome. What makes it uniquely different from other chronic and often fatal diseases, such as diabetes or hypertension, is the flood of emotions—hate, anger, fear, frustration, shame, and grief—that almost always propel us into behaviors and decisions that get in the way of finding help or of accepting the help that's offered. And centuries of public misperception and public intolerance have also made it difficult for people to seek help in the first place.

My goal is to silence the noise and dilute the confusion. In *Now What?* you will find insights into the mind of the alcoholic and addict and explanations as to why addiction is a family illness. You will learn what to do to help yourself if you're the one with a problem with alcohol or other drugs, or what to do to help the person you love if you're a family member, spouse or partner, or significant other. You'll find information about why addiction is a disease and why people with this disease need treatment. You'll also learn about treatment and what to do when you leave treatment to ensure ongoing sobriety. You'll gain insight into why it is easier to stop using than to stay stopped—and how "remission" from the disease of addiction is a lifelong process.

And finally, you will learn to value the importance of standing up and speaking out about addiction and recovery to the next generation—your own children and grandchildren.

The journey you're about to embark on is never easy, but it is essential. Thank you for letting me be your guide.

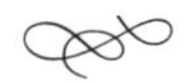

CHAPTER 1

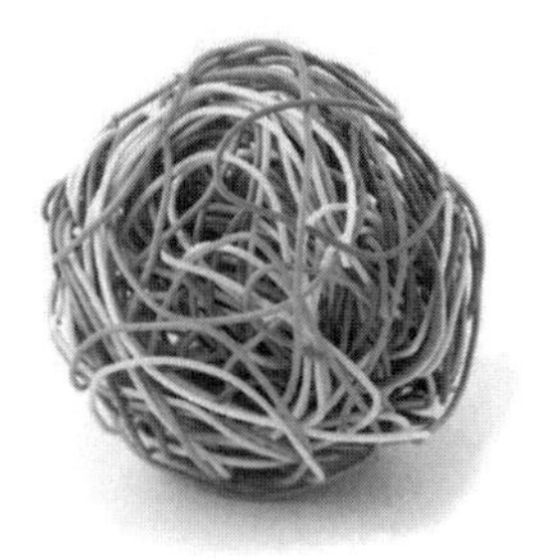

Swiss Cheese: The Addict's Brain on Drugs

"What's really happening inside the addict's brain?" probably isn't the first question that crosses somebody's mind when a spouse is caught driving drunk in a blackout or when a daughter sells her body on the street for a $20 rock of cocaine. It's more likely the person would ask in desperation, "*Why* would you *do* that?" But the question is never about what actually causes people to keep drinking or taking drugs to the detriment of everything that matters in their life, including life itself. The "Why?" is almost always a response to the bad things done by good people. Their immoral behavior when they know what's right and what's wrong. The complete disregard for the pain they're causing everyone they love.

"I mean, it's like the kitchen sink when she's drinking; she throws out everything that matters," an exasperated mother tells me, her metaphors as jumbled as her emotions. "I just don't get it."

Neither does the fiancée of a crack addict. "There are so many times that I don't understand him, so many times I want to just shake him and say, '*Don't you know what you're doing?*'"

Addicts looking for the next high almost always know what they're doing. But like their loved ones, they can't understand or explain *why* either. About as close as they come to even questioning their actions is when they desperately wonder why they do the same things over and over again, expecting different results.

"I'm having an out-of-body experience. I see it happening, I feel it happening, I wonder how it can be happening to me, but what's so odd is I still can't believe it's really me it's happening to," recalls a twenty-eight-year-old civil engineer and father of two children. "I say to myself, 'Come on, man, you should know better. What the hell are you thinking?'"

TRYING TO MAKE SENSE OF ADDICTION

Making sense of addiction is far from easy. In 2011, the American Society of Addiction Medicine (ASAM) updated its definition of addiction. On its website, its 3,000-word footnoted definition begins this way:

> Addiction is a primary, chronic disease of the brain reward, motivation, memory and related circuitry. Addiction affects neurotransmission and interactions within reward structures of the brain, including the nucleus accumbens, anterior cingulate cortex, basal forebrain, and amygdala, such that motivational hierarchies are altered and addictive behaviors, which may or may not include alcohol and other drug use, supplant healthy, self-care related behaviors. Addiction also affects neurotransmission and interactions between cortical and hippocampal circuits and brain reward structures, such that the memory of previous exposures to rewards (such as food, sex, alcohol and other drugs) leads to a biological and behavioral response to external cues, in turn triggering cravings and/or engagement in addictive behaviors.

Wow. Even I don't really get it, and that's my brain they're describing.

No wonder society still struggles to comprehend why addicts and alcoholics chase the dragon despite the merry-go-round consequences and to the detriment of all else that really matters in life.

No wonder those of us who have fought addiction in our own lives know it as "cunning, baffling, and powerful."

And no wonder that, after years of sobriety, relapse can inexplicably, suddenly erupt like a long-dormant volcano.

"My hope is that this definition will be very helpful for professionals and bring even more legitimacy to this misunderstood disease," said Dr. Marvin Seppala, a former ASAM board member and the chief medical officer at Hazelden, who knows firsthand about addiction, treatment, and recovery, both professionally and personally. "It helps those familiar with addiction and those who suffer with addiction come to an understanding that addictive behaviors and addictive thinking are the result of distinct alterations of brain functioning. Such recognition can relieve some of the shame and guilt that plagues those with addiction."

In 1987 the Partnership for a Drug-Free America launched a public service campaign to warn us about the dangerous effects of drugs on our bodies. Its public service announcement featured a close-up of a sizzling skillet on a stove. "This is drugs," the announcer said. An egg is cracked open into the skillet. "This is your brain on drugs," the announcer intoned. The twelve-second spot ended with the sound of the egg frying and a provocative, almost dismissive line: "Any questions?" *TV Guide* named it one of the top 100 commercials of all time. Decades later people still remember it, and last time I checked, almost a million people had viewed the campaign's PSAs as YouTube videos.

But the ad leaves the wrong impression that drugs fry the brain. They don't, any more than they stew, bake, broil, or steam it. To the contrary, what the ASAM definition tells us is that drugs baste and bathe the brain in its own pleasure-causing juices that are and have always been at the core of our cortexes.

CHASING DOPAMINE

In his voluminous history book *The Pursuit of Oblivion,* Richard Davenport-Hines chronicles 3,000 years of humankind's love affair with mood- and mind-altering substances. Ancient Egyptians had a cookbook with recipes for 700 opium concoctions. In the state of Georgia in the 1840s, "ether frolics" were popular. (When a doctor observed that people who injured themselves during these wild parties didn't seem to mind their pain, he experimented with the drug as a medical anesthetic.) Blot out the pain, alter reality, highlight the pleasure—the list is endless of ways our human species has pursued oblivion for good or ill by getting stoned or drunk or both.

"Intoxication is not unnatural or deviant," Davenport-Hines writes. Instead, he explains, we chase the high for all the right reasons, including "human perfectibility, the yearning for a perfect moment, the peace that comes from oblivion." He reports that F. Scott Fitzgerald, Marcel Proust, Edgar Allen Poe, and many other literary giants believed they did their best work under the influence of their drugs of choice. Even Bill Wilson, the cofounder of Alcoholics Anonymous (AA), spent the rest of his life looking for a way to re-create the powerful spiritual experience he had following the frightening aftereffects of his nearly fatal final drunk. The case can be made that the innate urge to feel better or just feel different never ends until we die.

It doesn't matter whether you're Bill Wilson, an Egyptian pharaoh, or a writer working on the great American novel, we humans habitually seek out what makes us feel loved, happy, and satisfied. All of us know pleasure when we have it and desire it when we don't. And although our hearts may flutter or beat faster with satisfaction, our brains tell us what feels good and remind us to come back for more. The most intricate of organs, the brain is where the body's "reward system" operates 24/7, releasing a naturally produced chemical called "dopamine" that is responsible for the pleasing, often euphoric effects of food, sex, and exercise. At one time or another, all of us have been under the influence of something that is highly pleasing. We get "high" when we eat something delicious, make love, run a marathon, or garner a bonus at work. Within a few hours, the dopamine level returns to a balanced or normal level and the brain goes on thinking and doing other things, until the next time. "Typically any reward that exceeds expectations releases dopamine," said Dr. Omar Manejwala, an addiction psychiatrist.

THE HIJACKED BRAIN

Alcohol and other drugs generate pleasingly copious levels of dopamine too. That's why we get loose and feel relaxed when we drink at the end of a hard day at work or after the kids are finally put to bed. Why we feel creatively energized by a line of cocaine. Why Vicodin makes a root canal worth it, and Valium loosens the grip of restless anxiety, stoking contentment. Dopamine does the job exactly as nature designed.

But when we drink enough alcohol or take enough of another mood-altering chemical, the amount of dopamine released is greater and unnaturally intense. Repeated intense exposure overloads the brain and eventually can burn out its delicately structured reward pathways, making the nerve cells' receptors less and less responsive to activities that would otherwise be a natural source of pleasure and joy. As the dopamine levels drop in the brains of addicts and alcoholics when they come down, they are propelled to keep taking more of the substances to increase their dopamine levels sufficiently to maintain the elusive euphoria. Robbed of free will, they find that getting high is no longer an optional pleasure: in the mind of the addict, it has become a matter of survival. The brain has been hijacked.

The brain is the organ we depend on for decision making, but a hijacked brain isn't going to make sound or rational choices. If we addicts make decisions based on the irrational belief that getting high is a matter of survival, then we'll do anything to keep experiencing the effect, whether it makes sense to the rest of the world or not. Alcoholics can find a cold beer in the desert. Addicts can find dry cocaine at the bottom of the ocean. A pill head can find one more Percocet in somebody else's medicine cabinet.

"The effect of such a powerful reward strongly motivates people to take drugs again and again," said Dr. Nora Volkow, the head of the National Institute on Drug Abuse, in a 2008 speech. "This is why scientists say that drug abuse is something we learn to do very, very well."

Yet every day millions of people drink responsibly. And millions of others occasionally use illegal drugs without major consequences. Many of them use substances to the point that they incur "teachable moments," incidents as serious as an arrest for driving under the influence, as minor as a misdemeanor charge for marijuana possession, or as simple as one too many hangovers. If so, they are apt to consciously modify their consumption, or quit altogether, to make sure those incidents don't happen again.

In college, my buddies partied like me, using the same types of drugs with the same frequency and even with some of the same negative outcomes. They all learned from these experiences, grew up, and moved on to focus on more important things, such as finding work, getting married, and starting a family. Only one of us—me—got hooked. Why, then, do such a small percentage of people who use substances develop a baffling inability to "just say no" and an addiction?

It turns out there's more to it than chasing dopamine. Ruben Baler, health scientist administrator at the National Institute on Drug Abuse, puts it this way:

> The influences that impact our brains can be seen as a stack of Swiss cheese slices. Each slice represents a different aspect of your life, with one slice standing for genetics, the adjacent one for brain development, and the next ones for early childhood experiences, family dynamics, the human-made environment, socioeconomic status, and so on. And, because this is Swiss cheese, each slice has different holes that correspond to specific risks—whether biological or environmental—that the "arrow" of substance abuse must traverse to become an addiction. Luckily, each slice also has many areas without holes (protective factors)

> with the ability to stop that arrow at any point in its trajectory.

No wonder people used to tell me I had a hole in my head! Long before we alcoholics and addicts ever took that first drink or drug, our brains were highly susceptible to all sorts of influences that make up the stack of Swiss cheese slices. Some slices we're born with, like the genetic entanglement of the deep roots of our family tree. Some are the microscopically intricate misfiring neurotransmitters we can't see. Others are the dominating monsters of sexual, emotional, and physical abuse that too many of us experienced. And even the environment we're living in right now has a role.

How the holes in these layers line up, or don't, is the deciding factor once our "arrow of substance abuse" enters the brain through that first high and onward. That's why intelligence is no more a bulwark against addiction than is brawn; it doesn't matter if you run a Fortune 500 company or pour concrete or are a stay-at-home parent. Nor is faith a protection: the most religious people can be just as vulnerable as atheists. Rich or poor, single or married, brilliant or average. These factors all come together in a dynamic that addiction professionals and neuroscientists understand now more than ever, but probably will never fully figure out.

Are some of us destined to become addicts from the get-go? There is compelling evidence for this outcome from pioneering studies involving twins.

Identical twins have identical genes. Twins born of addicted parents but raised in separate families—one in an alcoholic family, the other in a nonalcoholic family—both tend to become alcoholics themselves. But if the twins come from nonaddicted parents and one grows up in an alcoholic family while the other doesn't, neither twin typically develops addiction. In other words, genes matter when it comes to vulnerability to dependence on alcohol or other drugs.

"Essentially it comes down to nature *and* nurture," says Dr. Manejwala, echoing what many scientists and doctors now know about the internal and external dynamics of addiction. Both factors play significant roles.

So it's safe to say that it is all but impossible, short of solitary confinement or exile on a distant island, to completely shield somebody from the dynamics that can result in a full-blown addiction—some of us are just built and wired for it. Add to this societal and environmental factors, such as peer pressure, the social norms of alcohol and other drug use, and the overprescription of medications for what ails us, and the odds are stacked against a small percentage of people who are susceptible to the "perfect storm" of addiction. Public service campaigns, such as the fried egg in the skillet, or school programs like D.A.R.E. (Drug Abuse Resistance Education) aren't effective with those of us who are alcoholics and addicts, because simply scaring us or sheltering us from stoking our dopamine receptors is counter to our makeup. We use substances exactly because they do what we want. What we like. What we *need.* Right away. Now.

As she later told me, Marcy S. knew the odds:

> I have lived with this all of my life. My beloved grandmother, my dad who died from ulcers

> because of his drinking, my beautiful mother who used to dance me around the living room to *The Lawrence Welk Show* when I was little, my husband who had a heart of gold but no desire to stop drinking to take care of his sons, and now my son Scott, my beautiful son that I have tried so hard to protect. We have gained and lost everything over and over again.

Marcy's family heritage is rife with alcoholism. Her grandmother, mother, and husband all died as a result of their drinking. When she wrote to me "Help, my son is dying," she feared Scott was next.

"I'm a walking book on alcoholism and alcoholics," she said. "But knowing it and warning Scott about the risks weren't enough, I've realized. Children learn what they live."

I once met a woman who, precisely because of what she knew about her family's past, told me she had never taken a drink or a drug in her thirty-five years. Her motive was simple: "I feared the family tree. Everyone in my family is an alcoholic. The risk is just not worth it. I don't want to be one either." She was an exception until two years ago when she broke her leg while skiing. In the hospital, she was given a generous supply of pain medication by doctors who did not know her family history. "I discovered all the joys of a freedom like nothing I'd ever known, a purity of self and satisfaction beyond anything I had ever achieved of my own effort," she said. "Pandora's box was unlocked; out of it I floated above the old me to that blissful place, heaven." After a few weeks on the mend, it was time for her to come off the pain meds. "It was hell; I fought like hell for more, just one more," she said. "That's when I came face-to-face with the realization of what my family members themselves must have faced in their own addictions. Damn, I'd become just like them." No matter how hard she had tried, the odds were against her. The holes in her Swiss cheese lined up, too, and the arrow of prescription drugs pierced her core and exploded into addiction.

FILLING THE HOLE IN THE SOUL

If addiction were simply about the effect of dopamine on an oddly wired brain plus the holes in the layers of our own personal "cheese stacks," then brain surgeons and pharmaceutical companies probably would have cured it by now by filling in some of the holes. But there is another opening in the body of an addict that's got nothing to do with the head. I call it the "hole in the soul."

Everybody's got one. It is deep within each of us, where we yearn for fulfillment. And although dopamine doesn't go there, filling that void in the soul can have the same effect as dopamine on the brain's receptors. It feels good—not just the same "good" as sensual pleasure, but a deeper, longer-lasting "good" that nourishes the deeper part of ourselves. How do we "fill" that hole? Filling this hole is about finding our place in life and understanding what gives life meaning. We seek out all kinds of experiences essential to life's journey, such as our ever-evolving relationship with a Higher Power, a power greater than the small self of sense gratification that taking drugs fulfills. That power can be awakened any number of ways, from spiritual practices paying homage to the God of our understanding, to contemplating the glory of the changing seasons, to writing in a journal as a discipline to gain more self-awareness.

The hole in the addict's soul, in contrast, percolates with a throbbing sense of unhappiness, a restlessness, irritability, and discontent with life defined by feelings of inadequacy, of not fitting in. There's a feeling of not being good enough, of never being satisfied with who we are, usually based on our own impossible standards more than the expectations of others. A hole that is all about the pervasive sense of not measuring up, of imperfection stemming from our inability to come to grips with being flawed human beings like everybody else. "Do you know the impossible dilemma of having to be perfect in the body of a human being?" I often ask addicts. And they nod, because they know exactly what I mean.

These feelings are not unique to alcoholics. All humans suffer from varying degrees of not having enough of whatever satisfies the human spirit. What separates alcoholics from everyone else is how, unconsciously at first, they relieve this ache. Substances such as marijuana, opiates, or alcohol are our elixirs. And we usually discover this by accident, for although we may start out using them for the same reasons everybody else does, we soon discover that these substances medicate the pain in our soul and magically fill the void. Getting high is so easy—and it works! We don't have to try so hard anymore to be better or feel better. We become more tolerant of our own shortcomings. We don't itch so much anymore while living in our own skin. We become less sensitive to the people, places, and things that taunt us, especially those voices in our own heads.

That's why, even decades later, many alcoholics and addicts recall the epiphany of their first drink or drug.

An eighty-eight-year-old combat veteran of World War II, a man who had tasted bootlegger's home brew for the first time when he was thirteen, told me this:

> In my long life, I've seen plenty and experienced it all, just about, but today [one of] my most vivid memories remains of that moment. Recalling it even now I get that same warm, flooding sensation of peace and utter joy that flooded into my belly and rose like the high tide to my head that night. It was like a magic potion. Everything was okay with me. I was okay with me.

I, too, remember my first high. An older co-worker offered me his joint, and I accepted it mostly because I wanted to be part of the crowd. I really had no idea what to expect; I had never been buzzed before. But in the moments after the smoke filled my lungs, suddenly I became the teenager I wanted to be. I had arrived. And it had barely taken any effort. Dopamine pleasure flooded my entire body with a sensation I had never felt before. For as long as the buzz lingered, that pit in my stomach no longer ached. The rapture of the moment was so intense that I chased it for two decades and never forgot it.

Cheryl M. doesn't remember her first drink. She was only three years old. Her father was a successful brewmeister in St. Louis, and in their German family, a little beer at bedtime was not only a good sedative but was accepted as the proper way to say good night. Her father also was an alcoholic, and her mother suffered from tuberculosis. "As a child in an alcoholic family, I had lots of opportunities to experience depression and disempowerment—parents who were physically, mentally, and emotionally absent," she explained. "I was unhappy and desperate." Rather than filling a hole in her soul, booze replaced her soul as it faded away altogether.

"Alcohol gave me hope, it made me feel good, made me competent. I saw it as a solution, not the problem, because this is what made it possible to live life," she said. Yet she, like many alcoholics, discovered the impossibility of a life under the influence. Eventually, she ended up homeless and living in a shelter. It took eight treatments in four years before she finally stopped drinking. That was twenty-nine years ago. She's been sober since.

Cheryl's experiences and those of millions like her show that addiction is as much a suffering of the troubled spirit as it is a problem of flawed circuitry in the complicated layers of the brain. Yes, positron emission tomography (PET) scans clearly show the impact of substances on the brain. And studies on twins, as well as the commonality of stories of families like Marcy's, prove the genetic dynamic too. But what cannot be tangibly captured with the high-tech instruments of science or quantified with research using control groups is this soul-sickness endemic to everyone who becomes consumed by what they consume. The perpetual shifting between intense shame and the camouflage of delusional grandiosity common among addicts is grounded in perspectives that are inaccurate, incomplete, and, therefore, out of touch with reality. Addicts typically believe they deserve more than they have and, at the same time, think they don't deserve what they get. All along, addicts are convinced that life is essentially unfair or should be fairer. They get high because they're unhappy, and they get high when they're happy because they can never be happy enough.

SLIDING OFF COURSE

A friend of mine has a sister whose twenty-year addiction to marijuana and alcohol has all but exhausted the family. Like so many other loved ones who don't understand, my friend finds himself delving deeper in hopes of looking beyond his sister's behavior to what torments her inside. "I kind of get it about the brain's chemistry . . . but what is it that's screwed up her feelings about herself, about the world around her, and caused her intrepid restlessness?" He asks what anyone who loves an addict asks: "How do substances 'consume the soul,' and why?"

There are a million ways and no way to simply explain it, although many people have tried. But for me, Jim Nelson comes the closest. He's a renowned Christian ethicist and the author of *Thirst,* which reveals his journey from addiction into recovery in the context of his own spiritual upbringing and formal education. Jim said all of us are created with a deep "thirst" for a spiritual power or presence to give our lives meaning and worth. But only for addicts and alcoholics are substances quite effective in appearing to satisfy this craving for a Higher Power. Here's how he explained it:

> Beyond its genetic and biological components, addiction is a profoundly spiritual disease, but the spirituality of addiction is idolatry, the substitution of a lesser god (in this case a substance) for the Infinite One. Idolatry always gives false promises but never delivers authentic meaning and wholeness. Just the opposite. Addictive idolatries not only disappoint but deeply damage the person and all of his or her relationships. The seductive power of alcohol for the alcoholic—"cunning, baffling, powerful"—is the craving for a false god, a thirst that cannot be satisfied by the substance.

Mood-altering substances hijack the brain not only by short-circuiting this natural process of thirsting and searching, but by relentlessly and recklessly driving it forward and over the edge. They eventually steal the soul, tilting a person's moral compass away from society's fundamental expectations, rules, and values passed on from generation to generation. The feelings, thoughts, and actions of the addict collide with the "norms" of the rest of the world.

People start out using drugs to feel better. Some use them to the point that it hurts, so they cut back or quit. About one in ten users crosses the chasm where it is no longer about *liking* to use substances: it is about loving them blindly, sometimes to death. The cravings of the hurting soul's unsatisfied needs meld with the brain's cravings for more of what feels good. From this cataclysm emerges the addict.

When this happens, everyone but the addict is blindsided, because to them the person's addiction seems to come out of nowhere. Yet long before the crisis comes to a head and finally exposes the raw truth, most addicts have already developed a gnawing, slow-motion sense that their lives are sliding off course. We know things "aren't right." We feel "dis-eased." What's actually going wrong, though, perplexes us. To protect our right to continue to drink and use, we instinctively assume a defensive stance that pushes back against the truth or deflects the focus onto other people and circumstances. That way, we don't have to take responsibility for the problems our drinking and drug use are causing. We ignore and defiantly refuse to accept the fundamental problem: alcohol and other drugs have mastered our lives and undermined our power of choice.

This is called denial. It is an insidious feature of addiction, because it skews addicts' perspective, convincing them that they don't need help or that they are capable of fixing themselves without the support and guidance of other people, whether professionals, friends, or family. For an addict, denial is all about justifications, excuses, and vows, which sound like some of these likely familiar phrases:

"Life is so unfair."

"If only my husband would stop haranguing me."

"I only use cocaine on weekends."

"If I stay away from gin and tonic and only drink lite beer, I'll be okay."

"I got that DUI because the stupid cops stopped me for a broken headlight."

"I'll quit tomorrow."

The repetitive frequency of such sentiments is in direct proportion to the addict's increasingly desperate condition. Usually this denial is as formidable as a fortress wall, even when help is close or the end is near.

The first time I ever consciously considered the impact that my use of drugs was having on me was in 1988, after a three-day streak on crack cocaine. Lying in bed, exhausted but wide awake, unable to eat even though I was emaciated, and in jeopardy of losing everything, I stared at the ceiling when suddenly it occurred to me: "*If* I have a drug problem, someday I might need help." The emphasis was on "*If*." Heck, I wasn't in denial about my drug use; I used drugs. I wasn't in denial that drugs caused problems. I had problems. My denial was my inability to grasp that I could no longer control my use to avoid the repeated consequences that were burying me alive. And so I kept hiding and using and denying every single day for another year—until I got help, which I did only reluctantly.

Does any of this justify the addict's behavior? No. Addiction is not an excuse. Denial is no defense. "You do the crime, you do the time, whether you're stone-cold sober or stoned out of your mind," I tell people, usually in talks to addicts who have ended up incarcerated. This is a fact: people voluntarily choose to use substances. But this is also a fact: I've never met anyone who chose to become addicted. Any more than any parent has ever aspired to raise a child who is a heroin addict. Any more than somebody consciously sets out to marry an alcoholic.

Understanding these elements of the addict's mind, body, and spirit is crucial to what happens next, because the alternatives are simple: continuing to descend into the maelstrom of addiction or getting help. In the chapters ahead, we'll learn how addicted people who choose to get help can get better.

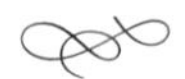

CHAPTER 2

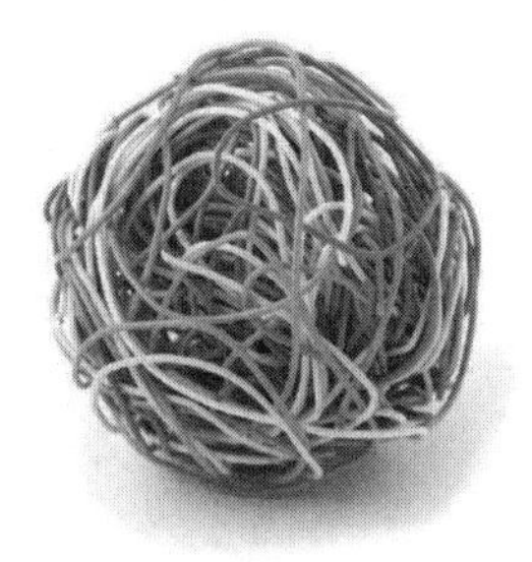

Bowling and Addiction

To understand addiction's impact, go to a bowling alley. Addiction is like bowling. The drug is the bowler. The addict is the ball. The lane is the addict's path. At the far end is a set of pins, which are all the elements that affect the addict's quality of life—physical health, mental health and emotional well-being, finances, employment, a role in the community, values and beliefs, and family. There goes the ball.

A wayward roll plunks the ball into the gutter. Once in the gutter, it stays there, the "chug-along" rumble building momentum as the ball's energy propels it onward. In a few seconds, it swooshes past the neatly placed pins, perhaps swirling the air just enough to sway them. But everything is left upright as the ball itself runs out of room against the back wall with a jarring thud. Just as suddenly, the ball drops out of sight and quietly disappears. But not for long.

Again the drug takes over. Automatically the ball returns to the bowler's hands. It spins down the lane again, out of control, and swerves into the gutter. Again and again and again the process repeats itself, the seemingly resilient ball always ending with a noticeable thud. But not for long.

After a while, the bowler, addiction, has put so much momentum behind the ball that it stays out of the gutter long enough to reach the inert and exposed pins, which are no match for what happens next. In ones, twos, or clusters, the pins are struck down with a violent force, unleashing enough energy to ricochet against each other. A few may remain upright while the stricken pins are swept aside. Sometimes they're even gathered up and restored to their previous spots. But not for long, because with enough rolls, eventually the drug delivers the consummate strike. Every pin is scattered helter-skelter. None are left standing.

Addiction is an illness that knocks asunder and blows away all the pins that matter to the addict or the addict's family. At one point or another—very probably right now, since you're reading this book—addiction has rocked you to the core. So let's take a quick inventory of some of the consequences a person incurs with addiction.

PHYSICAL HEALTH

Alcohol and other drugs make the addict sick with all kinds of physical problems that aren't typical in the average, healthy person: heart problems, skin rashes, sleeplessness, tremors or "shakes," jumpiness, ulcers, lethargy, hacking coughs, upset stomachs, rapid weight loss or gain, and a host of cognitive impairments. Eventually most alcoholics and addicts who don't get help are a physical mess. Amy, an addict three years into recovery, told me, "I got to the point pretty fast where I looked like I felt: a wreck. I just didn't care anymore."

These recurring symptoms evolve into related problems that are much more serious because the addict always gets worse, never better, as long as she keeps using. There are no exceptions. These more serious problems include chronic illnesses such as anemia, cirrhosis of the liver, or pancreatitis after sustained bouts of drinking. Hepatitis, herpes, and HIV/AIDS often are the direct result of the alcoholic's behaviors and choices. Addicts have a higher rate of death from cancer and heart attacks.

Perversely, as the addict's health consequences mount, the slide downward picks up speed because of the higher tolerance: the addict needs more and more of the drug to achieve the same effect. All the while his organs strain to keep up—until they can't. And then the body shuts down. Sometimes the damage is so severe it cannot be reversed, even after the addict recognizes the problem and seeks help. That's how baseball great Mickey Mantle died. Known for rowdy drunkenness during and after his playing days with the New York Yankees, he finally got treatment and got sober, but it was too late. Despite an eleventh-hour liver transplant, he had already drunk his body to death. He was only sixty-three years old. A year earlier, one of his sons, Billy, died of heart problems related to chronic drug use. He was thirty-six.

At a certain point in this excruciating process, only two alternatives remain for the addict: complete abstinence or sudden death. Abstinence is unlikely without a recovery program, which we'll devote most of the rest of this book to talking about. Sudden death can come in many ways: A heart attack when a jolt of cocaine interrupts the electromagnetic signals that make the heart beat in rhythm. A skull fractured in a bar fight. A bullet to the head on a street corner in a dope deal turned sour. A head-on collision from driving drunk the wrong way on a highway. Every day the obituaries are filled with such tragedies, although the stories rarely mention the addiction as the underlying cause of death. In my hometown, a community leader and respected businessman "died suddenly" at home before he turned fifty. In truth, he drank too much too often until one night he fell down the stairs and broke his neck. One of Hollywood's golden boys, William Holden, died in a similar way. He hit his head on a table and slowly bled to death because he was too drunk to call for help.

Traffic accidents are a leading cause of death due to drinking or drugging. Each year in the United States thousands of alcoholics die behind the wheel or kill others in traffic accidents. Even when multiple offenses are cited, though, seldom is the obvious likely true cause—alcoholism or other drug dependence—given its due.

On a summer Sunday afternoon Diane S., a thirty-six-year-old mother coming home from a weekend camping trip with her family, drove drunk and under the influence of marijuana. In her minivan were her own children and three nieces. For miles her van sped the wrong way on the Taconic Parkway near New York City before crashing into an oncoming vehicle. She died. So did her daughter and her three nieces, as well as three men in the other vehicle. The accident generated enormous nationwide attention in 2009, but the question of whether she was an alcoholic or addict who had needed treatment apparently didn't come up.

"Because we have never known Diane to be anything but a responsible and caring mother and aunt, this raises more questions than it provides answers for our family," her brother, whose three girls were among the dead, said in a news story. "Amidst all the uncertainty and speculation as to how and why this accident occurred, this is the absolute last thing that we ever would have expected."

This family isn't alone. Seldom do people who use substances or who love a substance user expect death to come calling. Don't get me wrong. The manifestations of addiction's physical symptoms, whether in violent, shocking suddenness or in an excruciatingly slow erosion of the body's ability to function, aren't always an in-your-face wake-up call. That's because, as sick as addicts become in the throes of their substance use, a perverse resiliency often shields their decline and fall. This "shielding" can occur to the point that physical subterfuge is as prevalent as the psychological denial that blinds addicts to the truth. Their outsides don't always match their insides.

Staring in the mirror, for example, you might say to yourself, "I look a bit tired around the eyes, maybe a little bloated in the cheeks, but I don't look so bad." A spouse sees the woman he loves all dressed up and ready to go out for a night on the town and tells her, "You're just as beautiful as ever." A teacher notes a drop in the straight A's of her best student, but still he comes to class every day smiling, hair combed and teeth brushed.

For every alcoholic or drug user who looks and feels like a wreck, many others don't, even though they, too, are addicts. For these people, the ramifications have turned their lives upside down, but not inside out for all to see. Yes, extra makeup, a sick day at work to catch up on our sleep, or a convincing excuse for the bloody nose and black eye cover our inconvenient truth.

But the truth is that looking the part isn't a prerequisite to be an addict. And if you have one of those especially resilient metabolisms that can seemingly bounce back from the worst binge-drinking time after time and start all over again, just give it time. The clock is ticking for you as well.

MENTAL HEALTH AND EMOTIONAL WELL-BEING

Mood-altering substances can make addicts feel or see things that aren't real or find themselves wrangling relentlessly with delusional thinking that seems to have a life of its own. They may feel as though they're going insane. Recovering addicts also use the term *insanity* to describe the kind of delusional thinking that protects their ability to keep using, such as "I can have just one drink or hit and stop."

When my chronic use of cocaine led to sudden, uncontrollable nosebleeds in the late 1980s, I tried to blame it on a robber who pistol-whipped me one night in New York City. I told that story so often and with such vivid detail that I actually started to believe it myself, even though there was utterly no truth to it.

"In the end, it didn't matter—fact or fiction, the truth or a lie, it was all the same gobbledygook—the world I survived in was one big never-never land," Tricia M. said in recalling her own outrageous cover stories.

In some cases, addicts' episodes of delusional thinking can take the forms of diagnosable mental disorders. Almost two-thirds of people addicted to substances also struggle with diagnosable mental illnesses. Consciously or not, they will self-medicate and discover temporary relief from these mental health disorders that "co-occur" with their substance dependence. So they keep using them, even when alcohol or other drugs begin to worsen their condition, sharpening the edge of anxiety, expanding the extremes of bipolar disorder, or deepening their depression to the point that separating one problem from another is like unraveling a giant ball of old, frayed string. It's all tangled together.

David W. returned from two combat tours in Iraq in 2008 to discover he didn't "fit in." He and his wife had a young daughter and had been contentedly married for ten years before he came home and discovered that he felt disconnected from his family. And when he couldn't find a steady job, he spent most of his days around their suburban house feeling restless and edgy. "It wasn't about being bored; I just couldn't relax and find joy in the simple things anymore, the things that mattered." At the Veterans Administration hospital, he was diagnosed with post-traumatic stress disorder and prescribed medication with therapy. "I didn't believe in that stuff," David said. "Alcohol was easier, because it worked better." Soon he couldn't stop drinking. "It got to the point I wanted to do it on my own," he said, "or not at all."

But trying to untangle addiction from mental illness without proper medical or psychological guidance becomes risky, because no addict stays high 24/7. Eventually, either tomorrow morning or next week or sometime down the road, the access to the mood-altering substances that have been masking the symptoms of the mental disorder is interrupted. What can follow are waves of anxiety and desperation that overtake the addict's fragile mind and cause confusion and desperation. Addicts are often birds of a feather when they're getting drunk or high, but afterward become islands as solitary as Alcatraz, keeping company only with the shame, grief, and fears that helped feed their addiction in the first place. At one time or another every addict ponders this conundrum: "Drugs: I can't live with them, and I can't live without them." Unless addicts reach a point where they consciously decide enough is enough and want to get well, most addicts dodge the conundrum by getting high again. And again.

Unfortunately, a few desperate souls don't see a way out of the vicious cycle and decide to end it all.

This happened to my friend Clark T. In 1992 he lost eight years of sobriety in a relapse and became so entangled in his problems that he could not get free, even with the assistance of his family and mental health professionals. In his garage, Clark crawled into the back of his car with the engine running and killed himself.

It has been estimated that as many as 50 percent of all suicides involve alcohol or other drugs, and well over 90 percent of people who commit suicide have a diagnosable mental illness.

FINANCES

Money never keeps pace with addiction. For addicts, the substance is the only currency with value. When they're not under the influence, alcoholics and addicts obsess about how to get that way, and that always requires cash.

Addiction among the Wealthy

The wealthiest addicts have it easier for a time, because getting high or staying high only requires they go to the ATM machine or write a check or "borrow" from their families. Usually that's not a crime, although I've known some conniving addicts whose proclivity to get at the family fortune is tantamount to extortion if not outright armed robbery. For the most part, wealthy addicts only steal from themselves to feed their craving and they have some left over to mitigate the consequences when it is time to pay off the drug dealer, post bail to get out of jail, hire a lawyer, make restitution, and get professional help or treatment—especially when they don't want their insurance company or others to know. Rich addicts usually have enough but always end up with less.

That's exactly what happened to one addict I worked with. Even after his family cut him off, he depleted twenty years of savings in his own 401(k) accounts, and nearly $1 million soon shrank to $19,000, still enough to get help one more time when he finally realized he was done using. Although he's been sober for six years now, he still laments, "I'll never get back what I lost. I worked as hard to lose it as I did in earning it."

Addiction among the Poor

Among the poor, addiction simply exacerbates poverty and pushes them deeper into the hole of economic despair. Poor addicts don't have the luxury of their wealthier counterparts' financial "problems." They just have the addiction problem. So they often resort to burglary, robbery, dealing drugs, and prostitution, often accompanied by violence, to make the money needed to feed their habit. And whatever money they make goes to the dealer or the liquor store with nothing left over for anything else.

I've known the poorest of addicts who'll barter food stamps from the wallets of their own families for an hour's worth of high. That's why so many poor addicts end up in jail, on the streets, or living in a shelter. Poor addicts don't start with much and they end up losing everything. That's what happened to everybody I hung with in the Atlanta crack house where I hit bottom in 1994. A few years after I got sober, I was lecturing to public health and social work students at Emory University, not far from that crack house, when a woman, herself a social worker, stood up at the back of the audience and interrupted me: "Mr. Moyers, our agency knew those people you were with in that crack house," she called out. "Most of them are dead now." Their desire to escape their addiction was no less than mine. I'm the only one who did, and only because I had insurance and other resources, including my family's support.

Addiction within the Middle Class

In between the rich and poor is everyone else, and in a way, they're the ones who perhaps know the toughest economic consequences of addiction. Middle-class addicts start out with something but can't hold on to what they have. That's because for most middle-class people it takes everything they've got to pay the utility bills and put food on the table, save for retirement, pay the mortgage or car loan, and set something aside for a child's college education. When addiction suddenly knocks them over, they are often trapped in a hellish catch-22. Their dilemma isn't too many options or none at all. They have choices, especially if they have health insurance. But the options are limited, and family members' desperate desire to give what it takes to help the addict get well often comes at the cost of meeting their other expenses. It is enough to drive families over the edge, and it often does.

One couple I know raised two sons in a hard-working two-income household in Michigan. With it came all the trappings of middle-class success. At the same moment the economy collapsed in 2008, their oldest son was gripped by addiction. Help required money they didn't have. The husband offered to trade his boat to a treatment center. His wife offered her wedding ring.

That's what happened to Marcy S. too. "I had resources, barely, to help Scott. What I quickly learned was the curse of knowing that it wasn't going to be enough if he didn't get better. Then what would I do?"

Whether you are rich, poor, or in between, addiction always takes and never gives back.

EMPLOYMENT

It is a myth that addiction mostly affects unemployed people. To the contrary, most addicts and alcoholics "function" at work—until they don't. Up to that moment they may be known for working hard, meeting tasks, and completing assignments, whether on the assembly line or in the corner office. But as the disease progresses, an addict can't keep up his increasing level of use for long and still manage to do a good job or keep the job without getting noticed.

Addiction is the ultimate "boss." Addiction is in charge, and the addict will go to any length to satisfy the ever-demanding pressures of keeping the boss happy. That is the only bottom line that matters for the addict, even if it means missing work, stealing from co-workers, or showing up at a meeting under the influence.

Eventually addiction almost always wins the tug-of-war between what an addict knows she must do to keep a job and what she cannot stop doing to risk losing it. Even her employer giving her one last chance doesn't keep her straight. "You're fired" is a consequence most addicts know at least once. Losing a vital job or derailing a promising career is sometimes the wake-up call an addict needs, but usually it only accelerates the downward spiral that eventually appears as gaps on a resumé.

COMMUNITY

Thank goodness the stereotype is long gone of the "town drunk," that benign, almost endearing lush of a character who once was as much a part of the community as the butcher, the baker, and the cops on the beat. The fact is that addiction is a disease of isolation, and although addicts may find a "community" among other drunks and users, they mostly become alienated from their nonusing friends and their larger community. Addicts will usually reach a point at which they no longer have time for friends because those relationships are forged and depend on personal dynamics and common interests that have been worn thin by the addicts' selfish obsession with maintaining their addiction.

Besides, an addict's friends seem to have an uncanny knack for sniffing out a problem long before anyone else—even family. The friends are more apt to speak up too. One person told me, "I lost my very best friend when I told her I didn't like what drugs and the people she was hanging with were doing to her. She got pissed and took off. . . . Eventually she did get help. She's still around town, but we haven't gotten together in years."

If the addict is a student, school becomes problematic, because attendance gauges participation and grades reflect performance. Addicts are not consistently good at either. I know of an honor student and varsity basketball player whose binge drinking wiped her out during her junior year in college. Her parents had no clue until her grades came during the holiday break. "They'd believe anything I told them, but I'm not a very good liar. I broke down and told them the truth the day after Christmas: I'm a drunk." That was a year ago. She has taken a leave of absence from school to get help but still struggles. She worried, "Right now I don't think I can go back."

Among churchgoing addicts, even the most religious are likely to eventually lapse. Not only does the fellowship of the spirit pale compared to the "higher power" of the substance, but a sanctuary filled with believers is a cruel reminder of a life gone astray and will only spur further remorse and self-flagellation.

Twenty-one years later, I still shudder about the time I went to Sunday service after an all-night cocaine binge. I was desperate to find a firm spot to steady myself in the midst of the dizzying spiral of my struggle. Instead I felt myself a secret contradiction to the piousness all around me. I couldn't wait to leave, and I didn't return to church until I got sober.

Addicts retreat from the life and community they once shared and end up living in the confining loneliness of their quiet desperation.

VALUES, BELIEFS, AND INTEGRITY

I believe in the inherent goodness of all people and that it comes from an essential set of values and beliefs that we are given with varying degrees of effectiveness by our families and community. No addict is born and raised without a toolbox of these values, although no two boxes are exactly the same size or contain the same tools. But we all carry in us some combination of values or beliefs—such as the importance of honesty, courage, a sense of justice, respect for accomplishment, and loyalty—to help us make sense of life and to cope with what's ahead.

I've never met an addict who didn't have a set of core beliefs and aspire to live those beliefs day to day. Among these addicts are some of the kindest, most sincere, and big-hearted people on earth who will give you a dime if you ask for a nickel or who will loan you their car even if all you want is a ride.

However, practicing addicts will act and behave in direct contradiction to their core essential values. They don't do as they want to do any more than they do as they say. They do what the drug compels them to, and the need to get high takes on a value of survival that can override all others.

I know a death-row inmate who killed two employees in a liquor store robbery in the early 1980s and had this to say:

> My mama raised me right. She taught me good, she told me the good I do will always be the good I am. Mama made me stay in school too . . . she cried big joyful tears on the day I graduated and joined the Navy. She was real proud of me 'cause she done me good and I done her good back. But I got this alcoholic "streak" runnin' through me. My drinking outran me 'till the day I wanted it so bad I just snapped. Shot 'em down over a damn case of beer and a fifth of Jack Daniels whiskey because they wouldn't give it up without a fight. Stupid. Damn, I knew it ain't right, but I did it anyway.

Most addicts don't end up killing people. But we all play hide-and-seek with the uncompromising demands of our addiction, resorting to lying, cheating, and pulling out all the stops to keep up with the diminishing returns of our incalculable investment in our illness. We give away what matters to selfishly grab what we need. We go so far as to pull up the floorboards of our foundation in a futile bid to shore up the soggy flanks of our lives as they fall apart. And still we sink deeper and deeper into the moralless pit now void of what matters the most: our own integrity and self-esteem.

I recall the times in the stifling summer of 1989 when I stopped to buy ice cream from a vendor for the nameless kids who played on the Harlem street corner below the run-down tenement building where I was smoking crack and drinking malt liquor. "Hey, Mister, you're a nice guy," the kids hooted and hollered as they crowded around me, the pied piper who appeared in their neighborhood. And I believed them, or wanted to, before I headed upstairs to add to the misery of their neighborhood. I was desperate to do something right to counter what I knew I was doing wrong.

It is one of the most cunning twists of this illness. So many of us drink or take drugs either to alleviate the pain of facing parts of ourselves that we don't like or to puff up the parts that we do like in a bid to make ourselves better than we are. Yet we end up destroying what we value and aspire to believe, that we are on earth to do good and to receive good, no matter our circumstances.

FAMILY

Unlike any other chronic illness, addiction tears apart families.

"I hate you," I recall my father saying, in the moment after an intervention in 1994 compelled me to walk out of a crack house on the last morning I was high. After multiple treatments and an equal number of relapses through the years, I could relate to his raw emotion.

"I hate me too," I replied.

Hate. Anger. Dismay. Frustration. Rage. Disappointment. Shame. Fear. These aren't sentiments hurled by, and at, the people with breast cancer or hypertension. Nobody is pissed off at the diabetic who goes into shock for missing an insulin injection or the parent with Parkinson's disease who can't feed himself because of unsteady hands. With most debilitating illnesses come empathy and sympathy, nurturing and unflinching support.

Not so with the sick addict, because addiction infects the family as much as it does the alcoholic or drug addict with the same raw emotions, jarring invectives, brutal lies, unhealthy behaviors, and ultimately, the same results. Everybody gets sick or sicker.

Why? Before the onset of the illness, in many families there exist dynamics that are fundamental to a healthy relationship, mainly love, trust, nurturing, and compassion. The relationships of our lives wouldn't matter if we didn't love each other. We wouldn't want to be together if sharing life's ups and downs weren't part of the journey. If we didn't care about each other, we wouldn't stay together; we couldn't if we didn't trust each other.

When addiction strikes, though, it damages every single member in a healthy family relationship and frays the ties that bind us. The addict can be sneaky, selfish, irresponsible, foolish, mean, unpredictable, and even dangerous. And who wants to live with, much less love, someone like that? Yet it is almost impossible to separate the addict's behaviors from the illness that causes those behaviors. Instead, the family is sucked into the vortex of the addict's tornadic, unpredictable existence. The family becomes damaged, hurt, and drained. Family members obsessively worry about the addict and what to do, so they don't focus on taking care of themselves. The addict's symptoms become their own. And just like the addict, they suffer physically, mentally, and emotionally. No wonder it is called a family disease.

A woman who came to me looking for help told me, "I've become part of him—I'm not doing the drugs, but I am living the addict." Not long after meeting the man of her life, she discovered his life included getting high on weekends, in her house. "I feel like a drug addict, like him. . . . I'm baffled about what to do because I love a drug addict," she said. "I feel helpless. I am watching him die right in front of me."

What makes it all worse is that addicts continue to refuse help even when it is offered. In physics it's called "magnetic repulsion" when two magnets' corresponding poles—positive to positive or negative to negative—are moved next to each other. The magnets push away and refuse to come together, no matter how hard they're pushed toward each other. I borrow the phrase, because this pushing away is a phenomenon unique to this illness, and a baffling one too. How can a family rally to the side of an addict when the addict won't stay by the family's side but instead runs away or hides, again and again and again?

I recall the first confrontation with my mother on a street corner in Harlem where I had been bingeing on cocaine for eight days in a row. "Please come home," she pleaded through her tears, her face wracked with fear. "No, no, I'm okay," I insisted, barely able to see or stand up straight. Two years later, relapsing in a drug house in St. Paul, I hid in a closet as my family, just feet away, desperately searched for me. Finally they left. I came out of hiding. I was relieved. Finally, I could get back to the only urge that mattered: chasing the high.

Denial isn't solely the addict's tendency. Denial also obscures the family's ability to recognize the truth. This is a peculiar barrier in addiction; often the addict's family doesn't see the problem for what it really is, because nobody wants to believe they live with or love somebody who is an addict. "I'm not the mother to a monster," a defiant mother told me, "am I?" No, not a monster. But the stigma of addiction, like the effects of the illness itself, fosters a perception that what's happening to the person we love cannot possibly be happening.

Or we look for other reasons that are easier to stomach. Flunking out of school is due to poor study habits, parents believe. A wife convinces herself that her husband sleeps all day on weekends because he works too hard. A man hopes that his partner's unpaid bills and overdrawn account are due to financial mismanagement. A mother prays her daughter has learned a lesson and won't drive drunk again after getting picked up by the cops. A son doesn't know what to believe when his father comes home from the bar and beats up his mother in the other room.

That these things occur doesn't automatically make the offender an addict. But families often fail to connect the dots because of a fear of what they'll see: the bigger picture of addiction. And so families suffer and strain to understand senseless behaviors. We tolerate what we shouldn't, to the detriment of our own well-being. We accept what we abhor, because we feel guilty about what we feel. Or we choose not to feel at all.

And when the truth is so close it becomes the shadow we cannot deny, some of us opt to absorb the addict's behaviors as our own. Here's an explanation from Marc Hertz, an addiction and family recovery specialist who steers addicts and those who love them into treatment and sobriety:

> We become as incapable of being fully in the relationship, any relationship, as the addict. We "attempt" to control the addict's using, and when that fails, as it always does, we become just as agitated and crabby. We even engage in our own brand of hiding and sneaking, going through cell phones, e-mails, cars, and rooms, trying to figure out what exactly is going on, searching for proof. The family becomes just as toxic to the relationship as the addict, because we have manifested the same symptoms!

Jennifer E. likens her brother's addiction to that of a robber. Here is what she wrote to him in the throes of his illness:

> I wonder, are you growing tired of the robber? It has taken everything from you . . . your home, your money, your will and self-respect, your health, your relationships, your happiness, everything

> that makes life worth living. The power of this thief is amazing and dangerous, yet we still leave the door open time and time again to let you in, and so we let it in too. With great excitement and anticipation, we wait for the thief to arrive and continue to pillage . . . to take everything valuable. Sometimes if we haven't seen the robber for a while, we even go into a frenzied search for it, looking everywhere, doing whatever it takes to find it and let it eat our body and soul too. Our friends and families try to stop the thief, and deep down we want to stop it too. But something inside keeps allowing it in, often without our consent yet even without our resistance. This robber is so powerful [that] I believe it takes a well-equipped army who knows the entire thief's tactics to help give us the strength and knowledge to battle this elusive enemy. We must accept that we can't fight it alone.

A great myth of addiction is that the robber or thief lurks only in unstable, dysfunctional families. Everybody knows at least one such family, if it isn't your own. Families split open by blatant physical violence or unspoken sexual abuse. Those traumatized by the unanswered "Why?" after a parent dies or leaves without an explanation or after a child runs away and disappears. Families in which the blame game explains mom's drinking with dad's mental illness or mom's carousing or dad's plunge into his bottle of pills. Families in which the incessant drive for perfection covers up the bitter sting of disappointment until nobody can breathe, because they're suffocating in silent shame. Families void of love, trust, honesty, and nurturing.

For these families, addiction isn't the only blow. It is the final blow.

But no family is immune, even those families in which there is financial security, loving parents, and open communication. Families always suffer from the addict's illness; some just suffer more. Only by recognizing the toll it takes, only by embracing what is happening, do we begin to finally understand what motivates and drives the person who's sick with addiction. Accepting this reality is a fundamental first step to getting help—not just for the addict, but for everyone in their life.

As we're about to learn in the next chapter, capturing the monster, corralling the thief, isn't easy. It can be done, though. Once you recognize the problem, it's essential that you take the next steps to do something about it.

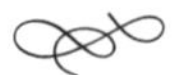

CHAPTER 3

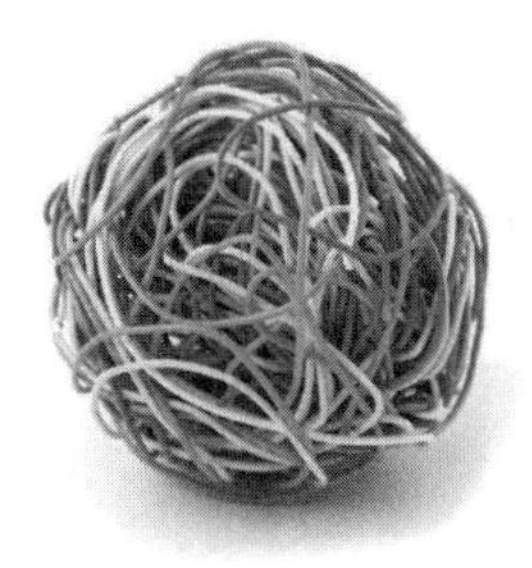

Giving Up by Giving In

Survival is a fundamental human instinct. A drowning woman fights tenaciously to keep her head above water. A child lost in a cave keeps moving toward the light, repeatedly calling out for help. A man trapped in the wreckage of a plane crash in a remote area lives on a single candy bar for days. When life is threatened, the will to survive takes over; life is all that matters.

This human instinct extends beyond those who are actually in dire straits. We don't go home to put on our bathing suit before we jump in to save the woman. We don't let our claustrophobia stop us from responding to a child's cry for help. When a plane crashes, our first reaction isn't to figure out whether it was caused by mechanical difficulties or weather. We do for others—friends, family, even strangers—what we expect them to do for us. To save a life in jeopardy. Right now.

A good example of this is a YouTube video of a 2011 accident scene that about a half-million people have watched. A motorcyclist is trapped under a burning car. Various passersby rush to the scene. Nobody is worried about how the accident occurred or the identity of the victim. They don't even know each other, but in seconds the crowd of Good Samaritans in unison lifts the vehicle off the roadway. The badly injured man is pulled to safety just in time.

A crisis doesn't have to involve a life-or-death decision to motivate us, either. When Alzheimer's or cancer affects a family, usually everybody rallies, putting aside their own priorities to help the afflicted. Neighborhoods have bake sales and block parties to raise money to offset a family's suddenly steep medical expenses. Churches hold prayer vigils. Friends adorn tree trunks with yellow ribbons of hope.

In my community, a woman with a failing kidney needed a transplant. An Internet website was set up, and willing donors quickly lined up for a possible match. Within a short time, the woman received the gift of a kidney from a college friend she hadn't seen in decades.

When it comes to each other, we are a compassionate, unselfish species in so many ways. But with alcoholism or drug dependence, our instincts often fail us.

When I meet patients in addiction treatment, I sometimes ask them, "Why did it take so darn long for you to get here?" Their furrowed brows or embarrassed chuckles reveal their truth. They don't really know. By the time they know they have to stop using and get help, they've usually racked up a long, expensive, and exacting list of consequences that they would never have tolerated or tried to endure if any other illness had caused them such pain.

When families exhausted by frustration and dismayed by their addict's behavior turn to me for help, usually they ask, "Should we wait for them to hit bottom?"

My reply: "Don't wait for them to die."

It is a dangerous, though popular, misconception that a sick addict can only quit using and start to get well when he "hits bottom," that is, reach a point at which he is desperate enough to willingly accept help. The ultimate bottom with addiction, however, is death. Anything short of death is an opportunity, perhaps the final opportunity or the final option, to overcome this fatal disease.

If you're the addict, consider this: Would you put off treatment for any other illness if you knew it might kill you at any moment? I doubt it. Would you want your family or friends to ignore your plight if they could help? Not likely. And as someone roiled by an addict's illness, would you turn your back if that person were seriously ill with any other life-threatening condition? No. Yet this is exactly what we do far too often, because it is impossible for addicts to see the truth—the very nature of their illness makes them incapable of making healthy decisions. They need help.

Yes, the addict has an illness, but one with a gamut of bizarre behaviors, unharnessed emotions, and perplexing consequences that are unlike those of any other illness. And one that gets worse until someone or something interrupts the chronic spiral toward that final "hitting bottom," death. And therein lies the most perplexing question with this chronic disease: short of the end of life, when is enough enough? The answer depends on whom you ask.

We'll look for the answer by learning about the lives of addicts who finally reached their breaking points without passing the point of no return. With the perspective of time, now they can look back with clarity and see how blind they were to the obvious decline and fall of their lives under the influence. "Duh, why didn't I get it any earlier?" is a standard question in most addicts' stories. And it is true: when the symptoms of addiction have progressed to the point at which the consequences are most devastating, short of death, it is shocking to realize how far and for how long somebody will go to keep getting high, rejecting the help they need, even when at some level they know how desperately they need it.

We'll also explore the quandary faced by people surrounding the addict or trapped in the addict's life. Their struggles to decide between doing everything and doing nothing, bouncing between the extremes of love and compassion and hate and disgust can bring them to their breaking points, hitting their "bottoms" as well. With luck, that bottom will bring them to the place where they can learn what it means to love that sick person even while letting them go. Addict, alcoholic, or loved one—we all suffer.

THE PROBLEM IS ME (FOR THE ADDICT)

You probably won't want to read this, but it is a fact: hitting bottom—that definable moment of jarring clarity that wakes up the addict to his predicament and finally separates that substance-warped illusion from the truth—can be a long time in coming. A long time measured in years. A long time measured in the runaway train of insufferable, unceasing consequences, often ignored even when they happen in rapid-fire succession. Such is the chronic condition of addiction, whether it suddenly grabs hold of kids in their teens or lingers for decades in older adults into the "golden years" of life.

Why is this? Because addicts believe they are in control. And for a while, their efforts can appear to be successful. We wait until payday to take a weekly jaunt to the crack house, convincing ourselves we won't spend it all to get high and will still have enough money to pay the bills. We binge-drink only on weekends, knowing we can sleep off the hangover on Sunday without shirking work and other responsibilities. We take a few extra pain meds in the comforting confines of our own living room, reassuring ourselves that we're not hurting anybody if all that happens is we bump into the furniture or nod off. We smoke dope at bedtime because it is the only way to get a good night's rest.

These aren't really excuses for drinking and drugging, because we don't need excuses to get high: we get high because we *have* to. We're merely justifying our "right" to get drunk or stoned by using our convoluted reasoning to show that we can control our use and its consequences.

"I started drinking because I liked it. It's pretty simple," recalls Scott S. "After a while alcohol got me into all kinds of trouble. That's when things got out of control, way, way overboard. It got to the point I'd never stop drinking until I ran out of money or was so screwed up and sick, and I'd swear 'Next time I won't let that happen again' and then it would, again and again."

We keep coming back to this justification among addicts in the early stages of their addiction. By qualifying or quantifying the use of the substance in the bigger picture of the rest of their lives, they can prove they're in control. Again, this works for a while. Many addicts will tell you that long before things got bad, they didn't see the cause and effect of their drug use precisely because life was manageable, if not downright good.

I know a Lutheran pastor whose leadership of his church gave him as much satisfaction as it did his parishioners. He was a spiritual presence in his Iowa farm community, revered for his selfless availability and tireless willingness to help people in need. He baptized babies, visited the sick at the hospital, and eulogized the dead. His Sunday sermons were works of art. For years he only drank to excess starting on Sunday afternoons, when he could let his collar down:

> I never drank just one or two. I usually got drunk, but alcohol never affected my reputation. I was a "closet" drinker. Alcohol relieved the stress of always being on call and having to be the perfect pastor in everyone else's eyes. As long as I could

> do my job and lead my church, that's the way I saw it; it wasn't a problem.

Years later he was treated for alcoholism and crack cocaine addiction.

In this way, addiction is like other health problems. The symptoms usually first show up when life is swimmingly fine, thank you. Either the problem isn't a big deal yet or people decide not to make it one. A mother with a dark, lumpy lesion may not think it is a problem, and besides, she's too busy raising her kids to get a doctor's opinion. That recurrent headache might be another migraine, or it might not. But as long as it passes, why not wait until later to get it checked out? Stress is causing those chest pains; stop worrying so much. We often practice procrastination caused by denial; most of us tend to put off for tomorrow what we should do today, especially when it comes to our own preventative health care.

Usually, though, at some point the obvious can't be ignored, and we realize that something is really wrong and requires the attention of medical experts. And then most sick people will do anything to get better. At that point, we usually don't look for any justification to avoid seeking help. We jump right in. We're worth it. We want to live.

Not so though when the symptoms are indicating the disease of addiction. Remember that no matter how much we appear to be in control of our use, or how good we are at justifying our continued use, we addicts get worse, never better. Remember that addiction is a progressive *disease* that involves increasing tolerance. We're always using more with greater frequency to climb that next higher peak to satisfy the craving. Occasional or episodic drinking and drugging isn't convenient anymore, nor is it possible, because it doesn't work. We start to use more of the time and then most of the time, setting new terms and conditions we could never have predicted. Why wait for payday to get high? Binge drinking doesn't know weekends. Pain meds work just as well on the job as they do at home. Marijuana enhances everything, not just sleep. A few belts of whiskey will improve my sermon, my sales pitch, my enjoyment of the party or of my daughter's graduation. And suddenly the addict is like the driver of a car on black ice. We've still got our hands on the wheel, grasping to keep our life pointed in the right direction. But the force of nature—the nature of the illness—has taken away our illusion of control. The addict slips and slides off course. (For a simple self-assessment tool to see if your symptoms meet the criteria for addiction, see appendix B.)

The futility of trying to control our use separates an addict from everybody else who uses mood- and mind-altering substances. With good reason, or for no reason at all, most people can stop or alter their use on their own when they choose to. We addicts can't do that, despite our best efforts. Our mind-set is all about maintaining access to, and control of, the substances. We lie, cheat, and steal with such skill that we convince ourselves we've got it figured out, and at the same time, we do our best to keep others from figuring us out.

This works until it doesn't, but when it fails we push on, shifting our energies to try to steer clear of the *onrushing* hazards and barriers, including the people who only want to help us but whom we perceive as standing in our way. The lying, cheating, and stealing continues to increasingly desperate lengths until finally nothing works anymore. Denial, which has worked so well at keeping us and those around us from seeing the truth, has finally failed us too!

By this time, at some level, we know the facts—we know that our lives are unmanageable and we know the reason is that our alcohol and other drug use is out of control. We see it. We fear it. We suffer it. We cannot escape it. And still, many of us are not quite done using.

My mentor, Bob, tells this story:

> An alcoholic stands before three doors. She opens the first door and an assailant with a sledgehammer jumps out and hits her on the head, knocking her to the ground. The door closes. Dazed, the woman gets up and opens the second door. The same thing happens. The assailant strikes. The pain is excruciating. The woman struggles to get up, makes her way to the third door and opens it. This time the assailant turns and runs, without attacking. So the woman chases after him.

What a hideous quandary. Once there was a time when these substances made us feel good and eased what ailed us. Now they are the cause of the pain that is our wrecked life. We're hit with it head-on. *The jig is up.* The meteorite has flamed out.

Maybe.

Because now fear takes over. Our brain shakes off the substances that have hijacked it long enough to engage the instinct that suddenly is our primary dilemma: fight or flight. We're at a crossroad. In this moment we can see only two options: make a run for it, or stand and face the phalanx charging to our rescue. For, if we're lucky, while we've been withdrawing into the darkness of our illness, some people may have been paying attention. And like it or not, we've got their attention. We sense their presence outside looking in, ready to take action.

We're intimate with some of them. They may include our spouses and partners, our parents, and our children. People who had sway over us, and we over them, through the love that binds us as the families we were before addiction swept us away. Others are our friends. They don't like what has happened to us. They're dismayed by the company we keep in drug dens and bars. If we've been fortunate enough to still be working, also crowding around us now may be bosses, colleagues at work, and the employee-assistance professionals who are giving us one more chance to keep our jobs. In the mix, too, may be the pastor of our church, our neighbors, our doctor, an attorney, and everyone else who is sick and tired of our shenanigans. Often the police are there, too, and a judge and prosecutor. We are surrounded.

THE PROBLEM IS YOU (FOR THE LOVED ONES OF THE ADDICT)

Oh, what an arduous, convoluted, and concentrated effort it takes to find the dots and to connect them to see the big picture. This is true with addiction more than with any other illness, for reasons that invariably begin with the addict's family. A unique characteristic of addiction is that the symptoms gripping the addict have counterparts among the people who love the addict. In the same way that addicts don't think they have a problem, justify their use, try to mitigate their circumstances, and dodge the truth, so, too, do their families. It's hard to believe, but true: often the family ends up as sick as the addict.

As an example, this is how Connie D. described her experience with her addicted thirty-four-year-old son:

> It was a long and painful process; I didn't want anything to do with it at first. I denied it, tried to act as if it wasn't there, like it wasn't happening to *me!* After all, I didn't deserve this; I wasn't an addict, not by any terms that I could wrap my mind around. *Why* couldn't he just stop it? This was embarrassing! *Just stop—just say no!* Well, he couldn't . . . and no amount of pleading or bargaining was going to make any difference *and* why was I so upset anyway? This is a disease.

Most parents don't want to believe their children have more than "a little problem with drugs." Maybe it is just a youthful aberration that will fade when they grow up. After all, everybody's doing it, and they're just trying to fit in, right?

Children also don't want to believe their parents can't stop getting high. Maybe dad will stop driving drunk now that he's been busted again. Or after all, mom has chronic pain and she really needs to take all that Oxycodone.

A wife can't imagine the person she married isn't the man whom she lives and sleeps with now. She hopes he'll quit pouring all the money into his cocaine use, and they'll go back to being like they were. Maybe he will finally pull it together if she threatens to leave him again, she thinks. Between the problem and the action to solve it there are plenty of plausible maybes.

For every hint that something's not right, it is very easy for the addict's family to look the other way by looking for an excuse ("It's all that stress at work—marijuana keeps me sane"), an explanation ("Everybody we know drinks a lot"), or worse, a perfectly logical reason not to take the next step ("If they find out he's a meth addict, he'll lose his job and we wouldn't be able to afford treatment"). Ignorance is neither bliss nor a defense. But it sure does obscure the truth about addiction, even when the facts stare you right in the face.

Through the decades—and especially since Melody Beattie first called it what it is, "co-dependency"—libraries of books have been written about the unique relationships between addicted people and their families. This entangling, enmeshed manifestation of addiction often obscures the clarity of perspective that is essential to take action to solve it. In lockstep with how addicts reach the point when they try to control their use, their families try to control the addict's behavior, usually with money, shelter, food, bail, pleas, tears, violence, and anger, to name just a few approaches—terms and conditions that rarely work, until the addict is ready. And as we know, addicts are never ready when we want them to be.

A codependent person is one who has let another person's behavior affect him or her, and who is obsessed with controlling that person's behavior.

The other person might be a child, an adult, a lover, a spouse, a brother, a sister, a grandparent, a parent, a client, or a best friend. He or she could be an alcoholic, a drug addict, a mentally or physically ill person, a normal person who occasionally has sad feelings. . . .

But the heart of the definition and recovery lies not in the other person—no matter how much we believe it does. It lies in ourselves, in the ways we have let other people's behavior affect us and in the ways we try to affect them: the obsessing, the controlling, the obsessive "helping," caretaking, low self-worth bordering on self-hatred, self-repression, abundance of anger and guilt, peculiar dependency on peculiar people, attraction to and tolerance for the bizarre other-centeredness that results in abandonment of self, communication problems, intimacy problems, and an ongoing whirlwind trip through the five-stage grief process.

—Melody Beattie, *Codependent No More*

At the same time, families are often told that the antidote to their own unhealthy behavior around the addict is to "let go and let God," embrace "powerlessness," just "stop enabling," and "set boundaries." These are solid as theories go. But as long as love is still part of the equation—and it usually is . . . why else would you stay in such a relationship for so long?—such counsel doesn't work for the family that hasn't had a lot of practice first. Who is ready to walk the fine line between enabling an addict's drug use and allowing him to fall and watching him die? Nobody I know—and I've been on both sides.

One man's approach, however, highlights what is possible—with practice. I featured him in a column I wrote called "Four Steps to Sanity." It is a good lesson for any of you who hate the illness infecting the person you love.

Four Steps to Sanity

The other day I had lunch with a man whose success in business has made him a lot of money. He is on the corporate boards of several Fortune 500 companies, rubs elbows with presidential candidates, dined with the Prince of Wales, and gets around on a private jet. The framed photos in his office captured it all.

He gives away a lot of money to provide health care for the working poor, to reform education, and to support his church.

But for the personal story he calmly shared, it would be easy to assume everything he touches turns

to gold. Not true; he has an adult child who struggles to overcome addiction. And no amount of love, compassion, persuasion, or financial support has resulted in his child remaining clean and sober for very long—at least not yet.

As parents like him know, his story is not unique. The family has been roiled by the child's addiction and hurtful, seemingly insane, behaviors followed by repeated, serious consequences. What struck me about his story is the clarity of practical action he has chosen to pursue in dealing with it. These are his four steps to sanity:

1. I LOVE MY CHILD.

"There is nothing more powerful than love, not even addiction. Love allows me to hold on to my daughter, to keep caring no matter what, while at the same time I can hate the illness that causes her and all of us such pain. With love there is no gap, no weak link, in my connection to my child."

2. I FORGIVE MY CHILD.

"It doesn't mean I condone her actions, but I know that with forgiveness I emasculate the power of addiction by separating the person I love from what the addiction is doing to that person and to the people who really care."

3. NEVER GIVE UP.

"Without hope, what do any of us have? Addiction wins if I just quit caring. Is that a message or the sentiment

I want my daughter to feel—that I don't care anymore? My door is always open. Closing it means I have no hope. Then what's left?"

4. TURN IT OVER TO A HIGHER POWER.

"Addiction tests my faith every day my child struggles, every time I feel the urgency to do something to save her. It is in those moments of utter powerlessness and despair that I have no practical choice but to find relief in my faith. Just knowing the presence of a Higher Power, even when I don't know the plan, relieves me of the heavy burden that it is up to me to save my child."

He smiled, telling me the story about the urgent family meeting called when his daughter had relapsed and disappeared again, leaving behind a disjointed trail of ATM withdrawals in the tough streets of a southern city, lies that punctured the family's close-knit fabric, and a terrified spouse with a baby.

"At the meeting I asked for a vote: 'Who is ready to have our Higher Power take it?' The vote was unanimous. That's all we could do."

He did something else too. "Every week I call and invite my daughter to dinner at our house." For months the invitations went unanswered. Then she showed up, quiet and withdrawn, "but there, with us," he said. "It's been a few months now. She fades in and out and disappears from our lives completely for a week . . . but on Sunday nights, the doorbell rings and in walks our daughter." About six months after he told me this story, his daughter was back in treatment again, desperate to recover, still trying, with hope. He helped her get there too.

No families can claim the ability to be a calming eye within the storm without making big mistakes, usually more than once. My family is among them. Yours probably is too. For too long we don't see the problem for the illness it is. Then we do, and in our instinct to rescue a life, we're so desperate to beat it back that we end up beating up each other and the addict too. To illustrate, Marcy S. recalled some of her and her son Scott's low points:

> Scott's little escapades, the wrecked car, being picked up for DUI, over and over again the consequences—I just became so very angry at Scott, very angry and hurt. I screamed, "After all I've done to keep you out of this, how can you go back into it?" I actually felt hatred for Scott, so mad I'd go days without talking to him. My anger was the biggest impact, maybe bigger than the alcohol and drugs.

WHAT FAMILIES CAN DO

So often in their desperation to save an addict who is not yet ready to be saved, the family's best intentions fail or go awry. Remember the "fight or flight" effect: it remains the strongest of influences as the addict nears the end of his run. Rarely is even the most thoughtful, well-intentioned, and well-planned attempt to help successful while the addict is in the throes of fear for his very survival. When a family member's concern, no matter how well intentioned or expressed, goes toe-to-toe against the brutality of the substances in their loved one's life, it almost always gets knocked out at least once, usually repeatedly. In this heavyweight fight, everyone is likely to be left bloodied and bruised, angry, frustrated, fractured, despairing, and exhausted. So, now what? Here are some things you can do to help.

Communicate

From the beginning and to the very end, do everything you can to keep the lines of communication intact between you and your addict. Don't turn your back or close the door on the sick addict, any more than you would somebody who is riddled with cancer, bedridden with a heart condition, or slipping away into Alzheimer's disease. Stay in touch and stay connected. You certainly will need to set some terms around illegal or disruptive behavior, but invite him to dinner, include her in family celebrations, meet him for coffee at a neutral site. Send cards on her birthday and holidays. Remind her that you're around and that you care.

And at the end of every communication, be it face-to-face, over the phone, or via e-mail or text, be sure to ask, "Do you want help?" Regardless of his response, if he responds at all, always sign off with this affirmation: "I'm here and I want to help you."

Above all, avoid threats. Remember that the mind of the desperate, fearful addict can't process your threat any better than it can a tearful, emotional plea. That mind is lost elsewhere, compromised and totally subsumed by the drugs and alcohol that have stripped it bare of logic, empathy, and essential understanding. But somehow and somewhere deep in the recesses of the addict's darkest places, there remains a kernel of awareness that help is possible, because you asked her if she wanted it, and that help is available, because you offered it. Or maybe it is not a kernel of awareness but simply hope.

No matter which, don't sever his lifeline to you. It is probably his only one. And when he suddenly reaches out and grabs it, he'll hold on to you.

Plan

Maintaining a lifeline doesn't mean you passively sit back, waiting for your addict to hit bottom, because we know what that means. Even as you quietly persevere in keeping connections to your loved one, you need a plan, a course of action, and resources. These resources should include a family therapist or addiction counselor to guide you through the emotional turmoil of the experience. Identify and check out reputable treatment or medical facilities whose staff have the expertise to treat the specific issues and dynamics involving your addict. Ask professionals or people at treatment facilities whether they do a formal assessment for when your loved one is ready to take that step. (For a simple self-assessment tool your loved one can take to see whether their symptoms meet the criteria for addiction, see appendix B.) Some of the best facilities may be closer than you think. Contact them, start the process for admissions, determine the cost and how it will be paid for. If health insurance is a resource, call and find out the coverage. And push back if you feel the insurance company should do more.

Consider an Intervention

Vernon Johnson, who pioneered the formal process for intervening to compel addicts to get help, posed the challenge faced by people doing an intervention by asking this question: "How do you help someone who doesn't want help?" It is a question that taunts and haunts every family I've encountered: they simply cannot intellectually comprehend or emotionally stomach the idea of failing to go to any length to save the person they love before it is too late.

A formal intervention is an option. This involves all willing people affected by the addiction, often with a professional interventionist, gathering together to confront an addict with the consequences of his use for themselves and everyone around him and to get him into treatment. Interventions can work. Many people, including me, have been plucked from the point of no return, because our families didn't give up on us after we'd given up on ourselves, and they hired a trained, experienced interventionist to get involved. A professional is unencumbered by the family dynamics that so often fan the flames of an addict's behavior and the family's reaction to it.

Wendy N. chuckles today, but it wasn't funny thirty-five years ago when she was on the receiving end of an intervention:

> Boy, was I angry. The last five people I wanted in a room together at one time were my husband, our daughter, my parents, and *me,* the combustible mix that we were. That day when I stumbled into my house, there they were, with Mr. Johnson, there to help me. He was the emcee, the referee; it diffused everyone's emotions and kept the situation under control. My family was able to tell me their concerns, what they wanted for me. I could hear what they had to say. Finally it all made

> sense. . . . The next day I was in treatment. That was the end.

There's a lot of misinformation about intervention, much of it fueled by the popular media. Even the term suggests a harsh, unpleasant confrontation. It isn't, and shouldn't be. *Love First* is how Jeff and Debra Jay prioritize the process in their book of the same title. (See appendix D for their advice on writing a letter to the addict as a part of the intervention process.) Recent developments in interventions emphasize the importance of compassion in the form of "tough love" that involves finally setting the terms and limits with the addict that have been so difficult for families to commit to until now.

Remember, though, that to protect her addiction, the mind of the addict or alcoholic hardens into an impregnable defiance that may reject a professional intervention at any time during the process, in the same way arrest, bankruptcy, divorce, or a visit to the emergency room may have temporarily disrupted her use but not been enough to end it. In other words, interventions don't always work, or they don't always work when the family wants. Spurned, it isn't easy for the family not to give up. Don't. Keep connected, even if only from a distance.

Avoid Enabling

Keep in mind that staying connected doesn't mean you condone his ongoing drinking and drugging. Tell him you know exactly what he's doing and you don't like it. Don't facilitate his using either:

- Never lend money or a car to an addict.
- Don't allow him to use alcohol or illegal substances in your home.
- Don't make excuses or cover for her when she doesn't show up for work or school.
- Set rules and limits and be clear what you expect of him when and if he chooses to be in your company.
- And stick to those rules!

This is as much for your sake as it is for hers. An addict who thinks she can get away with it will always try to get away with it. Don't enable her into thinking she'll always be able to outsmart you to find a way to use and keep the status quo.

Help Yourself

So, stay connected, make your personalized plan, and then do this: take care of yourself.

I always remind families that, whether or not their addict stops using and starts to get well, the family deserves and needs to recover. Of course, this is always easier when the addict has finally come in from the wasteland of the illness. But as we know, this rarely happens in lockstep with your own struggle along the way. And unfortunately, sometimes it never happens, because some addicts do die.

People are often perplexed when I tell them, "Take care of you, because in the end, you are the only person you can take care of." I recommend families attend programs at treatment centers designed for them, even if their addict is still "out there." Attend church groups to strengthen faith, meditation circles to foster serenity. Take care of all of your whole self—mind, body, and spirit. This isn't easy—but it is essential. Addiction fosters helplessness and hopelessness. You counter it by staying connected to your addict, setting boundaries, having a plan, and taking care of yourself.

For tens of thousands, self-care means going to Al-Anon meetings (www.al-anon.alateen.org). Al-Anon is a peer Twelve Step recovery program for the loved ones of alcoholics (addicts' loved ones are welcome as well), where they share their experiences and learn how to apply the program to their individual situations.

By staying connected, offering help, refusing to enable, and taking care of yourself, you'll experience the empowerment of knowing you've done everything possible. You're ready for what comes next, no matter what.

GIVING IN, NOT GIVING UP

As we learned in chapter 1, addicts and alcoholics remember their first drink or drug, and in the same way, most of them recall their last. The "last drink" is a defining epiphany in our stories. With vividness and clarity, we liken it to a bolt of lightning, the parting of the Red Sea, a booming voice out of nowhere, or for some of us, a gentle whisper in the ear when we're flat on our backs. Many put it this way: "I got tired of being sick and tired." In that moment, at the "fight or flight" crossroad for the umpteenth time, suddenly we are aware there is another option. We don't have to run. We don't have to fight. We really can stop using.

Theologians, psychologists, philosophers, scientists, and moralists have all tried to explain how and why this happens. In his classic work *The Varieties of Religious Experience,* Lecture IX, William James came close in this passage on dealing with what he calls "undesirable affections," to which I will add the addict's obsession with drinking and using:

> There are only two ways in which it is possible to get rid of anger, worry, fear, despair, or other undesirable affections. One is that an opposite affection should overpoweringly break over us and the other is by getting so exhausted with the struggle that we have to stop—so we drop down, give up, and don't care any longer. Our emotional brain-centres strike work and we lapse into a temporary apathy. . . . So long as the egoistic worry of the sick soul guards the door, the expansive confidence of the soul of faith gains no presence. But let the former faint away, even but for a moment, and the latter can profit by the opportunity, and, having once acquired possession, may retain it.

A variety of probable and possible reasons exist, but among those of us who know this surrender experience firsthand, it really doesn't matter whether the experience results from our fried brain, leaks out from the suffering soul, or envelops us from a Power outside of ourselves. And you don't have to be religious to experience it, although among nonbelievers, this moment of release can be as close to a spiritual experience as they've ever had. What counts is that the moment happens and that we hold on to it. I call it hope.

Although the source of this experience remains a mystery, what has led up to it isn't. For now the consequences of our lives under the influence touch us like never before, and for the first time, we're struck by our utterly futile attempts to change on our own the course that our lives have taken up to this very moment. Despite every good intention, the mistakes of the past, and our resolve to change, here we are again in a big mess. We are powerless over the substances, yes, but not defenseless.

There is a misconception that addicts don't have any influence over their decision to stop using. We do, in the same way that people with other chronic illnesses can choose to become part of the solution. With these illnesses, such as diabetes, hypertension, or Crohn's disease, we don't question that we have a disease, that we need outside help if we want to learn to manage the symptoms. In the case of addiction, though, we cannot get well until we understand that we are sick—sick with an illness we can't control, much less recover from, as long as we keep feeding it. The choice to treat the disease then becomes ours.

"We all stop at exactly the same point, when we finally decide to put down the shovel we've used to dig ourselves a deeper hole," said Mike S., who has been clean and sober for more than thirty years. He sought help when he was still young, twenty-six, with no legal, medical, financial, family, or employment problems:

> In my case, it was about reaching that point where I realized my drinking was out of control, and when I heard other alcoholics' stories I compared myself and said, "Yes, I did that," or "I could have done that," or "Thank God I never did that."

The same is true for Cookie J.:

> My consequences were relatively minor, but the toll on my psyche was quite significant. I did see how [drinking] was affecting my life, my children, my marriage. I was a binger, not an everyday drinker. But I was a poor mother on those hangover days, and I finally recognized it, which is what drove me to seek help. I realize there are many types of druggies and alcoholics, but I do think we are all able to see what we are doing to ourselves and others and, therefore, we are responsible.

For some addicts, like Mike and Cookie, the prospect of what might happen next is what finally wakes them up. For others the wake-up comes from the reality of something that has just happened. A woman in my community knew she had a drinking problem before she killed somebody as she drove herself home from a high school graduation party. She got help, but only after a life was lost. A star high school athlete had several alcohol-related scrapes before he turned eighteen, and he still managed to get a full scholarship to a Big Ten football program. Then he kept drinking and was kicked off the team, lost his scholarship, and dropped out. He returned to college only after he got sober, two decades later. Our prisons are packed with people who now understand what got them there. Some wake-up calls come early. Some arrive late, often at the expense of our victims. The victims or their families argue that it is too late, and often for them it is. Many times it is too late for everyone except us. We still have a last chance.

Mine occurred in 1994, after a cocaine binge drove me to my knees in an Atlanta crack house. I was thirty-five, and the craving was so intense that what I knew I shouldn't do was exactly what I did. I got high, and then I kept getting high even as my community tried to figure out how to save me from my illness. They had plenty of experience. Their efforts had always compelled me to seek treatment, but I still hadn't grasped the pervasiveness of my problem or my inability to dictate my own outcome by controlling it. And so all of what others did for me was for naught. There I was—again. At the same damn crossroad, only worse than ever before. I couldn't run. I couldn't fight.

Then on that October morning a simple question popped into my exhausted head: "Now what?" For the first time in my long struggle with this illness, I couldn't answer the question. In that moment I realized I couldn't do it anymore on my own. "Help me," I said to nobody in particular. I saw another way to go, and I walked out of the crack house and into the arms of the people who couldn't make me stop, but who were prepared and waiting for me when I was ready for rescue. I've been clean ever since.

For all of us, recovery begins the moment our inside world matches the outside world, and reality and perception become one. "It takes great courage to surrender," a general once told his troops. For us, it does too. Because surrender isn't about giving up. That would be easy: just kill ourselves or keep using until we die. Instead, we give in because we're done fighting. We don't care about getting high anymore. We care about living. So we give in and accept the help that is necessary to move beyond this moment, without ever forgetting the importance of this moment.

I'd like to close this chapter with Bill H.'s story that he told in *Undrunk*, the book he wrote under the pen name A. J. Adams, published by Hazelden in 2009. It sums up everything I've said so far.

> There is good medical evidence that alcoholism is a progressive disease. At the end, it progressed at a dizzying speed for me. Even though I was the one doing the drinking, I saw myself as the victim—of my wife, my boss, the doctor and shrink who were trying to help me, even my own children, who were frightened by what I had become and tried to avoid me. I was increasingly afraid of my unpredictability. I was so toxic that whenever my blood alcohol level dropped down anywhere near normal, I felt as though I was going to have a heart attack. My memories of this period are sketchy.
>
> After a few months of this final spiral, I found myself in county detox on a Friday and in rehab

two days later. My reaction to being in rehab was towering anger. Fortunately, my wife did not cave in to my demands to come home. After some early rebellion, including being late for everything and grinding on the nurses for more Librium, something strange started to happen. It began to dawn on me that "beating" rehab would be the emptiest of victories. I had spent years retreating from sobriety. Every time I felt the pressure to get straight, I made a concession or two—like cutting down or even going on the wagon for awhile—and then went back to drinking as usual. In the military they call this "defense in depth." You keep dropping back to what you hope will be a more defensible position—but you are still retreating. When I finally walked into an AA meeting, I wasn't there to quit drinking. I was there to *keep* drinking. After a few days in rehab, it started to sink in that this wasn't going to be my ticket to a few more months of drinking; it was probably my last chance to quit. That thought really scared me, so I ignored it.

As I look back, I think three things had to happen to give me a second chance. First, I had to understand that vital parts of my life were coming unglued. I had to feel genuine pain. I was not yet a shipwreck, but the trend lines were unmistakable. Second, I had to accept that my problem was alcohol. It was not this person or that one. It was not this unfair situation or that missed opportunity. It was booze. Third, I had to accept that I could not moderate my drinking. Every first drink led to a bunch more, no matter how good my intentions. I had to understand that getting this monkey off my back was not something I could do on my own.

After a week or so—and in spite of myself—I started to listen. Other people were clearly beginning to get it, and I wanted to get it, too. They say that "AA moves at the speed of pain," and my pain in those first days was increasing as I realized that this might be my last opportunity to save my ass. The next part is either spooky or magical. I'm not sure exactly why, but my mind opened a crack to what was being said, and my listening turned to hearing. Months later I would understand that what came over me was willingness. Willingness to accept my alcoholism. Willingness to accept help. Willingness to work the recovery program. Willingness to save my own life. I have to admit, this made everything that followed a lot easier.

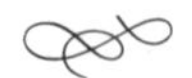

CHAPTER 4

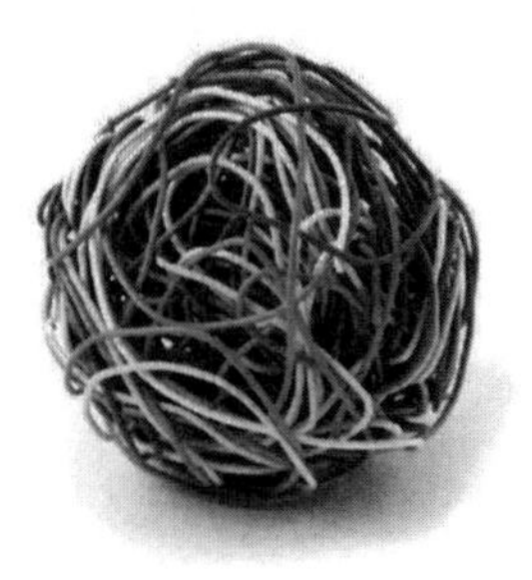

Treatment

Let's clear this up right now: treatment is not a prerequisite to surviving addiction.

That's a bold proclamation, coming from a guy like me. I required four intense treatment experiences over five years before I finally put down the alcohol and other drugs. I'm biased by default, too, because my employer, the Hazelden Foundation, is a leader in providing addiction treatment, and since 1949, thousands of people like me have found assistance at Hazelden. Many thousands more have done the same at treatment programs all over the country.

So yes, treatment works to make recovery possible. But recovery is also possible without treatment, especially after 1939 when *Alcoholics Anonymous* was published and the Twelve Step peer-recovery movement became a national phenomenon. For the thousands of years that people have been using mood-altering chemicals, there are those people who, out of options and in baffled desperation, have found enough reasons to quit, whether through an epiphany in church, a wake-up call from a DUI, a stint behind bars, or a chance attendance at or an invitation to their first Twelve Step meeting. I know many old-timers who were never patients in a treatment center.

Louis Zamperini's larger-than-life story (featured in *Unbroken,* Laura Hillenbrand's 2010 biography) is a prime example. A 1936 Olympic runner, Zamperini survived being lost at sea during World War II and then endured brutal years as a prisoner of the Japanese. After the war, he drank to excess to cope with what we now call post-traumatic stress disorder. In the 1950s, he suddenly stopped his drinking after having an epiphany during a tent revival put on by evangelist Billy Graham.

What worked for Zamperini and others is what still works today, no matter how they do it or at what point in their lives. I call it "spontaneous remission," and whether it happens with no warning or after an avalanche of consequences, what matters is that it happens and you hold on to it. Here's how Marne S. recalled her spontaneous remission:

> I got out of high school and dropped out of college pretty quick because my alcohol was my whole

> life. I was all of like twenty years old when one day I woke up and didn't remember what happened last night. Lying in bed next to a guy who'd vomited all over himself, a guy I vaguely knew . . . it occurred to me, "This is not acceptable; this is not working." I said out loud, "That's it. No more."

With a throbbing hangover, she stumbled into the kitchen, washed down four aspirin with a shot of vodka, poured the rest of the bottle down the drain, and hasn't had a drop of alcohol since. That was five years ago. Today she's a successful artist and new mother of twins.

As we know from earlier chapters, usually nothing works until the addict or alcoholic is beaten down, ready to quit being part of the problem and begin to consciously invest in the solution with personal responsibility first and foremost. For better or worse, it's that simple. As long as death doesn't overtake us, recovery always remains an option. And that's the point at which treatment can play a key role, because it is during the treatment process that we begin to fully grasp the potent nature of what ails us. In treatment, we learn our lonely perspective isn't exclusively our own. We start to learn what it takes to help ourselves. We begin to absorb and believe the possibilities of something beyond our plight right now. We start to prepare for what's next, the rest of our lives.

The term *treatment* has come to be shorthand for a formal program of intervention, assessment, education, and therapy designed to interrupt the downward spiral of compulsive alcohol and drug use and to give the addict the tools to stay sober and drug-free. As I tell patients, treatment ruins your "using" experience, because it usually shatters, once if not for all time, the illusion of control. "Would you really opt for treatment," I ask patients, "if you could control when and how much you drink?" Of course not, because treatment takes time, money, effort. Besides, treatment isn't meant to be fun (although it isn't unusual to hear people during treatment or as they are leaving say that it's been the most positive and rewarding experience in their lives). People who seek treatment usually do so because their lives are a mess, or heading that way, despite their Herculean efforts to affect the course on their own.

I'm a layperson, not a counselor or clinician, and someone who has personally experienced treatment as a patient. Although my life today is a direct result of the effective clinically based treatment I received in 1989, 1991, and after three years of sobriety followed by a relapse, twice in 1994, I am not an expert on treatment programs or which will be the best one for you. What I needed and what worked for me isn't necessarily what you or your loved one require, but here's some basic information I've pulled together from the experts to help you understand what's available.

TREATMENT OPTIONS

Today more than 14,000 specialized facilities in the United States treat addiction-related problems. No two are exactly the same, even when the facilities practice the same approach. The best way to find what kinds of programs are available is to ask for a recommendation from a mental health or addictions counselor or a medical professional whom you trust.

You may have friends or colleagues you can turn to who have been in treatment or have had family members in a program. If this doesn't work, you can go to the Substance Abuse and Mental Health Services Administration (SAMHSA) website, http://findtreatment.samhsa.gov. Click where indicated to enter the Treatment Facility Locator, and then click on your state and provide some basic information to find a licensed facility.

When a person contacts a treatment center, before admitting someone, all reputable centers will do a full assessment of the person to determine whether he or she meets the criteria for substance dependence (see the Diagnostic Criteria sidebar). Included in the pre-admittance assessment will also be a battery of tests for co-occurring mental disorders, such as depression, anxiety, or personality disorders. Treatment centers, whether inpatient or outpatient, should have mental health professionals available to treat these disorders, including a psychiatrist or other medical doctor who can prescribe medication as needed. Research is showing that it's ideal to treat both the addiction and the mental disorders in the same place at the same time, which is an approach called "integrated treatment."

Most treatment programs will support a Twelve Step abstinence-based approach, meaning they will require complete abstinence from alcohol and other drugs and will recommend attendance in a peer support group such as Alcoholics Anonymous or Narcotics Anonymous.

Programming differs from facility to facility but generally includes group sessions in which clients talk about their experiences, lectures on addiction and recovery science and

DIAGNOSTIC CRITERIA FOR SUBSTANCE DEPENDENCE

Alcoholism and other drug addictions fall under the category of substance dependence in the *Diagnostic and Statistical Manual of Mental Disorders* (DSM-IV): the recognized reference guide published by the American Psychiatric Association for psychiatrists, psychologists, social workers, addiction counselors, and other mental health professionals. This list shows the diagnostic criteria for substance dependence (three or more in a twelve-month period qualifies as dependence):

- tolerance (marked increase in amount; marked decrease in effect)
- characteristic withdrawal symptoms; substance taken to relieve withdrawal
- substance taken in larger amount and for longer period than intended
- persistent desire or repeated unsuccessful attempt to quit
- much time/activity to obtain, use, recover
- important social, occupational, or recreational activities given up or reduced
- use continues despite knowledge of adverse consequences (for example, failure to fulfill role obligation, use when physically hazardous)

Source: American Psychiatric Association, *Diagnostic and Statistical Manual of Mental Disorders*, 4th. ed., Text Revision (Washington, DC: American Psychiatric Association, 2000). Note: These criteria may be revised in the manual's forthcoming fifth edition, to be published in 2013.

practices, physical exercise and therapy, nutritional and spiritual counseling, and mental health counseling as needed. Most facilities have a family program in which spouses and other key family members join the addicts to learn about recovery and to participate in group sessions to prepare for those in treatment to come home.

Almost all of these programs offer aftercare and recovery management guidance—for example, AIDS counseling and medication management, methadone maintenance for heroin addicts, and job counseling. The most common aftercare program supported by just about all of the treatment programs mentioned is going to AA, NA, or another Twelve Step peer-support group regularly and working a Twelve Step program. We'll talk more about that in chapter 5.

In general, abstinence-oriented treatment falls under four categories: residential or inpatient, outpatient, private counseling, and jail or prison treatment. Let's look at each category more closely.

Residential or Inpatient

With inpatient treatment, you live, sleep, eat, and breathe the experience, because this is where you are 24/7, usually for a month or longer, depending on the severity of your condition. The facility may be freestanding or in the wing of a hospital or other medical facility. It is licensed to provide specific addiction treatment, which means insurance coverage is likely to include part or most of the cost. This is often the most expensive form of treatment, due to the length of stay, the cost of room and board, and generally more staff, which include the variety of professionals needed to address all the medical, psychological, and spiritual needs of the clients. The treatment center is equipped with, or has access to, a supervised detoxification regimen to safeguard the patient from the aftershocks of stopping and to address related health problems.

Main Advantages

There is more time, a variety of services available, and an intensity of programming in which you focus on nothing but getting well, sharing the intimacy of the experiences that landed you there with a lot of other alcoholics and addicts who are looking for healing from the same disease. Depending on the severity of your addiction and the attendant medical and psychological problems, inpatient treatment may be the only option for providing the services needed.

Main Disadvantages

You have to leave your job, your family, and the familiarity of the comforts of home for the time you're an inpatient. Also the expense is higher than for other treatment categories.

Outpatient

Outpatient treatment sessions, including group and some individual therapy, happen several times a week, generally for four or more weeks. These sessions usually occur in the evenings after work and on weekends, but sometimes are held during the day. About 80 percent of all treatment is now provided as outpatient services, which can be provided in treatment facilities, social services agencies, storefronts, or mental health clinics. Most outpatient services are licensed and are covered by insurance. The cost is less than for inpatient treatment, because there is no room and board and the programming is less intensive with fewer staff, although intensive outpatient programs can offer programming very similar to that of an inpatient unit.

Main Advantages

You sleep in your own room at home, keep going to work, interact with your family, and don't eat institutional fare. Outpatient services are usually less expensive than other treatment categories.

Main Disadvantages

Life is a distraction and can be an arduous challenge when you first put down the substances you were using and try to deal with life on *your* terms. The frayed family dynamic is all around you, and all the feelings and behaviors that your using instigated may still be there, even if the alcohol and drugs aren't. Your favorite watering hole, drug dealer, crack house, and the liquor cabinet are right where you left them the day before you started outpatient treatment. You might even pass them on the way to or from your treatment sessions.

Private Counseling

For those who can afford it or whose insurance will pay, psychiatrists, psychologists, social workers, addiction counselors, and clergy who have a specialty in addiction treatment will work one-on-one to help you get well. Sessions are usually held in their offices one or more times per week. Consider the counselor your very own concierge to recovery, except that a lot more is at stake than just a reservation at a prime restaurant or theater tickets. Many competent counselors are available, but it's important that you find a board-certified, licensed professional in counseling that includes addiction.

Main Advantages

You get undivided attention in the convenient and private setting of a nice office.

Main Disadvantages

You're all by yourself, and you miss out on the interaction and support of a bunch of newly minted recovering women and men—a group to affirm that you don't have to be alone anymore or to do it by yourself. The cost can be high compared with other treatments.

Jail or Prison

If your drug and alcohol use has landed you behind bars, believe it or not, good treatment is available for inmates in some states and in federal prisons. Treatment includes therapeutic communities, a long-term program with stringent rules and expectations (starting with living drug-free) set down and enforced by participants who are supervised by trained staff. Having access to such programs is the challenge; usually these programs have a waiting list and limited financing, with many programs being cut when state funding disappears. More than 75 percent of inmates are imprisoned because of a crime directly related to their alcohol or other drug use, although not all those inmates are addicted. Drug courts, which postpone sentencing pending completion of mandated treatment, can be very effective in compelling defendants to get clean, while also reducing inmate overcrowding and the chances of returning to crime.

Main Advantages

You can turn a bad situation into an opportunity for real rehabilitation and come out of jail or prison in better shape than you were when you went in, which usually can't be said for inmates who are not in such a program.

Main Disadvantages

Some criminals in prison have the goal to become better criminals, and they continue their addict or dealer lifestyle. (So if you still can get help before things get this bad, do it.)

SELECTING THE RIGHT PROGRAM

The challenge is selecting the program that matches your needs or those of the person you love. So how do you do this?

It depends on how you've reached this point. Usually the realization of the need for treatment is the result of a crisis. That's what happened in this family:

> A lot of personal relationships were badly bruised in the initial days of facing the reality of our son's addiction, because we did not know where to turn. Our longtime respected doctors did not know, our wonderful pastor could only pray with us, [and] the stigma of 1989 prevented us from asking friends for help. Reeling from the shock of discovering the depth of our beloved's illness, we failed to find help for several weeks. Only when I reached out to a very close friend and my husband reached out to an intimate friend who was a physician in

> another state did we begin to comprehend the possibility of recovery for ourselves and our son. Looking back on our own experience, I wish that we had known of a sort of 911 number to call when our family was confronted with the facts that our beloved son and brother was seriously sick with addiction. Now, more than twenty-two years later, we are all better informed about addiction and we believe in recovery because of experience and good access to treatment services. Now we know that the triage approach at the end of an 800-number help line might have provided the information we desperately needed.

That's my mother Judith's recollection—and I come from a family that has always prided itself on knowing what to do about a lot of things, or where to start looking when we don't know. When I suddenly reappeared from a crack house after eight days removed from the rest of the world, though, my parents were as clueless as any other family is likely to be. Few families contemplate addiction hitting so close to home. It's just not a topic of conversation around the dinner table.

Admittedly, things have improved since my family's time. Two decades ago, the SAMSHA treatment locator website wasn't available, and many medical professionals weren't knowledgeable about addiction, much less about which treatment programs would work best. Getting recommendations from friends was problematic for the same reasons, not to mention the stigma still attached to addiction back then.

Even with more resources and information readily available now, selecting a quality treatment program really starts by knowing what you or your loved one wants or needs. Usually this means first figuring out exactly what's going on. Of course it's obvious that alcohol or other drugs are the big problem. But what else is in play? Factors such as co-occurring mental illnesses, traumatic or physical disabilities, socioeconomic influences, cultural issues, or family dynamics can complicate and exacerbate addiction. Those complicating factors are why it is so important to get a thorough assessment, if possible, before you decide where to go for help. In an assessment, a trained professional asks questions and gathers information to make a comprehensive determination of the problems the addict is facing and how best to address them. Many assessments can be done with an appointment at local mental health or social service agencies or with private practitioners such as psychiatrists or psychologists. As mentioned earlier, most treatment programs also offer assessments before admittance, so you can start there, whether you ultimately use that program for the actual treatment or decide to go elsewhere.

Start the selection process by calling the different places that have been recommended or that you've identified in your research. Most treatment programs are waiting for your call with real human beings on the other end of the line who know what they're talking about, because people like you call them all the time with the same questions. You don't even have to identify yourself; just tell them you are interested in treatment options. It is imperative, though, to give them a complete picture of your circumstances, including the history of the problem, your insurance carrier, the addict's living and work situation and other special circumstances, and the person's related physical or mental health issues. If you don't already have these details based on an assessment, some facilities are even set up to do an assessment long distance.

Most addicts can't or don't want to go very far for help. In this day and age, especially when it comes to outpatient treatment, you may have several options in your community or nearby. So it might be possible to set up an appointment to meet with a staffer or, more importantly, somebody else who has been through the treatment and knows firsthand what it is like. Some treatment facilities connect alumni or parents with people in need in the community where they are located. Don't be shy about asking for that connection. There is nothing like hearing from somebody who has been there, has done that, and is on the road of recovery. Don't be deterred, though, if you cannot find the resources close to home. Sometimes, gaining distance from the milieu in which your drinking and using has occurred can be helpful.

In fact, "Don't be deterred" is good advice no matter the circumstances. Persistence may be needed to keep looking until an appropriate option is found, as Marcy S. describes regarding her son Scott's situation:

> After Scott hit bottom, I had him at our local hospital. The doctor said, "I'm sorry, but there is nothing else we can do for him here; there is nothing I can offer you in [Ohio]." Then the social

> worker walked in and said, "There's nothing we can do for this boy." I'd already been searching for something elsewhere, but the price, my goodness! They wanted thousands of dollars, and I just didn't have it. I got on the Internet again and kept looking for information, this time from other addicts, and finally I found a memoir—an addict's own story that was Scott's story, our story. I wrote the author a letter. That's when I learned of the option I never knew about, and Scott finally got what he needed, what I could finally afford.

Usually the scramble to find treatment options occurs in the same space and at the same time that the addict's out-of-control illness peaks, or nearly bottoms out, depending on your perspective. That means you, the addict or the loved one, are preoccupied. Don't be shy. It's an illness, and you can't deal with it by yourself any more than you should. Ask for help. Ask for help again. Keep asking for help—from family, the doctor, a trusted friend, a caseworker, an expert on the other end of the phone or e-mail, a pastor, or if you're lucky, a person in recovery. But keep asking somebody beyond the voice in your own head.

As an example, here's thirty-year-old Nic T.'s experience:

> I started using drugs again the day after I made bail. By the time my court date came up, I was right back where I started, no, worse. I told my lawyer I'd been getting high. "Don't say anything,"

> he advised me. Next thing I knew I'm in front of the judge, and it just came out, "Your honor, I'm a drug addict, I need help, I don't want to live like this anymore." The whole court got quiet. The judge looks up and says, "Your honesty is your new beginning, starting right now." He sentenced me to a year in the workhouse but put it off until I finished county drug treatment for [first-time misdemeanor] offenders. That was two years ago. I never went to jail. I'm still clean. It sure ain't easy. Sure beats the alternative.

Nic T., Marcy S., my family—nobody discovered the answer without asking for help. Once we get help, it is crucial to understand what being in treatment means, and what it doesn't. People's expectations and the impressions of treatment vary and those expectations and impressions must be addressed, too, for treatment to go smoothly.

FIVE COMMON MYTHS ABOUT TREATMENT

What are the most common myths and misperceptions about addiction treatment? Let's look at five of them.

Myth 1: Treatment fixes people.

All the time people implore me to do what this mother desired: "Just fix my son and send him home like the son I know, without the drugs." Nobody seeks treatment expecting less than to get completely well. By "well," they usually mean never again experiencing the inevitable, uncontrollable consequences caused by drinking and drugging too much. That's a fine goal. And this happens to many people; from the moment they start treatment, they leave the substances behind for good. But as we know, addiction is a chronic illness, meaning that it can be treated and managed with all sorts of therapies, including medications. However, addiction cannot—at least not yet and despite claims to the contrary—be "cured" or eradicated in the same way that a broken leg is repaired, a tumor is removed, or an infection is countered with antibiotics.

This is why addiction is so often compared to more chronic conditions, such as asthma, diabetes, cancer, or hypertension. The dynamics are treatable. Manageable. Always lurking. Rarely eliminated. A cornerstone of recovery is laid in treatment with abstinence as a goal. But the pervasive complexities of addiction include a mind prone to craving, a body that is allergic to what the brain desires, and a soul yearning for the elusive elixer to fill its hole. These factors are present before, during, and after an addict gets help. Treatment addresses the immediacy of the crisis by interrupting the pattern of use and offering the addict an alternative. It gives the person a chance to pause from the downward spiral. It helps him understand what's happening and his role in the problem and in the solution. It provides tools to find and maintain sobriety. It gives exhausted, stressed family members the same chance to catch their breath, find relief from the fear and chaos of the moment, and shift their focus to their own needs and wants.

Myth 2: Treatment brainwashes people.

Treatment is like graduating from school: you know more at graduation than when you started. So yes, addicts and alcoholics are never the same after they've been exposed to treatment, because they're smarter about their problems and wiser about the solution and what's at stake. This affects their thinking, and rare is the addict who doesn't get at least a glimpse of the impact their illness has in the larger context of their whole lives and what recovery offers to change that course.

But treatment doesn't seek to nor does it inexorably change the personalities that make each of us unique. Treatment doesn't deny history or erase past memories, good or bad, even as it helps to heal bruised consciousness and to sharpen a dulled conscience. It doesn't try to convert somebody into a follower of any secret belief system.

Most people come out of treatment with their religion of choice intact, if they had religion at all. But they do often emerge with a keen awareness of some sort of faith in a Higher Power beyond themselves and the potent power of the substances that whipped them. They still love their families, their hobbies, their pets, and whatever else made them the unique people they are. The best and the worst traits are still ingredients of their humanness. The only brainwashing was from the substances, so I guess you can say treatment is a kind of *de*programming.

Myth 3: Treatment is too expensive.

I hear this line all the time. My response is "Compared to what?" Compared to the cost of the substances, the price of the consequences? Life? The toll on society? The expense of the time well spent? The value of the result? I understand the source of some of this reaction. To this day there is a deeply entrenched sense among some people that alcoholics and addicts should be able to quit by themselves. "Go to church and be a better person." "Get some willpower and put your life in order." "Pay the court fine and buck up." "Just say no." All those approaches are free!

And that is why the sticker shock of treatment costs jolts people; they want a new car but not at the price of a new car. And until they suddenly shop for it, most people don't usually consider the cost, much less put money aside. Most people's rainy day funds don't include money for addiction treatment down the road. But for every seaside "resort" offering all the spa-like luxuries of treatment at $100,000 a month, most residential facilities charge prices affordable to the middle class. Many programs for the poor are free, supported with donations and public funding. Outpatient treatment is a fraction of the cost of inpatient treatment. And insurance companies are becoming more willing to treat addiction and mental illness like physical illnesses, especially with the parity law now coming into effect. (Passed by Congress and signed by then President Bush in 2008, the law bars most health insurance plans from unfairly restricting coverage, including financial and treatment options, for people seeking help for addiction and mental illness.) No matter what route you pursue, do it with the same vigor you would in figuring out how to pay for another serious or life-threatening illness. This includes engaging and standing firm with your health care insurer in finding solutions, and if the insurer pushes back, challenging the company to step up and follow the law.

Myth 4: Treatment doesn't work.

Yes, it does. "Our studies show that the 'compliance' rates for addiction treatment are at least equal to similar outcomes for diabetes, hypertension, and type 2 diabetes," notes Dr. Tom McLellan, CEO of Treatment Research Institute, citing his 2000 study published in the *Journal of the American Medical Association* comparing outcome data for addiction and these other chronic illness. In other words, the prospects for recovery from any of these illnesses are about the same. Yet people are often shocked when I tell them about Hazelden's track record: about 55 percent of our patients report they are still clean and sober in the year after they leave treatment. "That's all?" is the typical response. Again, to overcome this chronic illness requires the patient to actively engage in the treatment process.

And consider this: what is your definition of failure? If somebody finishes treatment, stays sober, and relapses two years later, does that mean treatment failed? Most people who relapse and go back into treatment or return to their Twelve Step program eventually recover. You can ask, but be wary of any program that claims a 100 percent success rate. There is no such thing. It's likely the program making such claims doesn't follow up with patients after discharge.

Myth 5: Miracles happen in treatment.

No, because if recovery were all about miracles, there would be no need for treatment. There would be no reason for trained counselors and experienced therapists and stringent regulations or licensing. No use for medication. No need for health insurance.

Granted, the organization I work for, Hazelden, was once called the "House of Miracles." I think I know why people believed it then and still call it a miracle when somebody recovers from addiction. It is because miracles happen when we least expect them. Or worse, the miracles happen when we've lost all hope for any other recourse. That's the point addicts reach just before they get well. That's what their loved ones believe too. Miracles seemingly happen against the laws of nature, and nature dictates that the human body, like the human spirit, collapses and dies when overcome by alcohol or other drugs.

But treatment doesn't defy nature. Treatment embraces nature by recognizing that addicted people suffer from a real illness that can be stopped and then healed with stringent processes, professionalism, dignity, respect, and compassion. "Miracles are not contrary to nature, but only contrary to what we know about nature," said St. Augustine.

Most important, miracles require nothing from those who receive them. Treatment, in contrast, demands hard effort, especially from those who benefit: the patients. People don't ever get well until they want to, and only then when they don't try to do it their way. Now is the time. I invite you to commit to the effort, to take the steps to get help for yourself or the one you love. Still hesitant? Then consider these personal messages to you, the addict, or you, the person in that addict's life.

An Open Letter to You, the Addict

Dear ____________________,

Either you know already or your family knows that you need help. This truth makes possible what occurs next: getting help. I am not a clinician, and thus any professional advice I give you is just that—advice, tempered by the reality that I don't know the mental, physical, and emotional particulars of your situation. Only doctors, counselors, and therapists, along with you and your loved ones, can determine with certainty what is vital to your next steps and, ultimately, to your ability to overcome what has driven you to this point. Now the goal here is to move beyond this point to treatment and, ultimately, along a pathway to wellness.

I do know good clinical treatment through my affiliation at Hazelden. I'm also aware of numerous local and national resources that can be tapped to assist you in your desire to get help. And as you know if you've read this far, I am the beneficiary of outstanding clinical expertise, given my four treatments over five years, my personal setbacks, and the emotional and spiritual growth I've experienced since 1994 when I finally recovered. Since I stood where you are now, nothing I've experienced in my own life could have happened without recovery as a constant goal. So I come to you mainly as a guy who's been there and done that, in more ways than one, and who now has opted to not get drunk or stoned again, one day at a time.

What about you? My hunch is you can relate. Otherwise you wouldn't have read this far and want to know more. You need help, although you might not yet quite grasp the seriousness of the problem. You want help, even if you're not sure what help looks like. You want to get healthier, although it's impossible for you to really appreciate what will happen once you do. You're at that damn crossroad—maybe for the first or third or tenth time—and not sure which way to go.

Only you will decide what to do. Finances, timing, work, your family, and legal consequences will all influence your decision. But whether you believe it or not right now, ultimately it will be self-will, yours and nobody else's, that affects what happens. If you try to dictate the terms and conditions—no matter how noble and justified they seem—then your prospects shrink. Your self-will did nothing to prevent your illness from unraveling your life. It can't put your life back together, either—at least not by itself.

If you convert self-will into determination, though, your prospects improve. You become determined to survive what's killing you. Now anchor that determination in accepting the truth that you don't really know what's best when it comes to treatment of your illness. How could you, any more than you would for any other serious, deadly illness? Others do know, however. They are professionals, experts in the treatment of addiction, and "fellow travelers" who are or have been right where you are. From this point forward, their collective experiences are invaluable. You must be determined to listen to them. Follow their lead and embrace their counsel. Use your determination to work diligently to put into practice what they teach you. Employ determination that keeps you coming back day after day after week after month, no matter what else affects your life or taunts your willingness to accept help until your treatment is complete. It's tough, but your determination will give you the perseverance you will rely on to trust the process and see it through. This isn't about following blindly. It is about keeping your head and your heart wide open to accept everything that goes into these early days, and ultimately for a lifetime, on the other side of your last drink or drug. Some of these challenges may seem too big to bear, others too trivial to bother with. Ignore neither; embrace both with determination that becomes a quiet conviction that there is a reason for everything that's happening.

Your self-will meant nothing to your ability to stop using. Your determination means everything to what happens next.

Treatment works if you work ***with*** *it, not against it.*

An Open Letter to You, the Loved One

Dear ______________________,

By now you're either furious and at wit's end or you're relieved and wondering what's next—or all of the above. In any case, you're no doubt exhausted. No wonder. What an effort you've poured into finding help for your loved one. You've repeatedly pushed, tugged, cajoled, connived, and otherwise run through the arsenal of your war chest to convince this important person in your life that the illness of addiction is destroying the person and you, all at once. You never fathomed how difficult this has proved to be. And although you've likely made mistakes along the way, you've also done a lot right and have made it this far intact. A wide gulf separates denial from acceptance, and bridging it demanded that you overcome the defiance of ignorance, fearful uncertainty, and the quandary of trying to love somebody with a disease you hate. Getting to this point is among the toughest challenges you've ever faced.

But here you are. Now your loved one is in a safer place, if not a better spot. Or the person is not, having escaped your grasp and fallen back into the clutches of a drug of choice. In either case, say it out loud: "I've done my part to help—for now."

Now it is your turn. Give yourself permission to step back and take care of yourself. You already know how to do this: gardening, church, exercise, a long nap, a weekend at the lake, a good book, or a string of home-cooked meals with your best friends around the table.

Now you must add one or two more salves to heal the wounds you can feel but cannot see. Get professional therapeutic counsel, and find the collective camaraderie of people just like you. If your loved one is in a facility that includes a family program component, go. If your efforts didn't get him or her into treatment, you can still go. And you should, because the program is for **you,** *not for the addict or alcoholic in your life. Find an Al-Anon group that includes people who know they must heal regardless of their loved one's journey—a regular group of old-timers and novices who remind each other they didn't* **cause,** *won't* **control,** *and can't* **cure** *their loved one's sickness. People who are at various points in their own journeys but are exactly where you are in the moment can remind you that you deserve to take care of yourself, and they will help you discover how.*

In one form or another I've passed along these messages to hundreds of people, their families, and others through the years. If my advice sounds like a cheerleader's "rah-rah" or a general's call to arms before the grand charge, then you haven't been where we are. By this time the struggle isn't about the problem or what to do about it. It is the addict's attitude that has become as critical to what happens next as the substances. It stands between now and what's next. Unaltered, the addict's closed belief system that fosters a myopic self-reliance and self-knowledge dooms the person to failure no matter where treatment occurs. Reformatted and redirected, this kind of resolve can actually become a tremendous asset.

Addicts work hard to get high or stay high. Convince them that their "work ethic" is worth applying to something else and they're apt to work just as hard to recover—except that now they won't be working in the solitary confinement of their illness.

This attitude is crucial to the treatment process. It becomes even more so later on. Treatment isn't the end. It is just the beginning.

A PERSONAL POSTSCRIPT

Effective treatment comes in many forms. What works for one person might not work for another, because there are so many pathways to get and stay sober and drug-free. But I want to make a personal case for what is probably the most widely applied and successful approach to addiction treatment and recovery: the Twelve Steps of Alcoholics Anonymous.

I know, some of you may be rolling your eyes, in part because the organization where I work founded the Minnesota Model that has the Twelve Steps at its foundation. "How can he be impartial and objective?" you're asking yourself or yelling aloud to nobody in particular but everyone within earshot.

Let me respond by setting the record straight. I'm not impartial. I can't be. This proved to be the model that finally got me—and tens of thousands of people like me—sober and drug-free. In fact, I'm ending this chapter about treatment with a column titled "It Works" that I wrote in August 2010 defending Twelve Step–based treatment from a critic. As they say in the Twelve Step program, "Take what works and leave the rest."

It Works

Why is there no debate about the effectiveness of Twelve Step–based treatment programs from addicts and alcoholics who have recovered?

Because for them, it works.

In [August] 2010, Bankole A. Johnson, chairman of the Department of Psychiatry and Neurobehavioral Sciences at the University of Virginia, garnered national media attention for his claims that treatment doesn't work and that even Alcoholics Anonymous is largely ineffective. Dr. Johnson argued that there is no real data proving most people get well. And he spit in the face of Twelve Step programs, calling them "weak medicine."

This from a doctor whose practice appears to treat addicts and alcoholics with medications, ignoring the reality that addiction is not only an illness affecting the mind but also the body and the spirit.

There is no doubt that the addiction treatment field has done a poor job of collecting long-term outcome data for patients. Alcoholics Anonymous, which is not treatment but is a recovery program that began in 1935 and today thrives around the world, has had a hard time gathering such data too. After all, its members are anonymous, so what numbers do exist are self-reported.

But in claiming that treatment is "ruinously expensive" and doesn't work, Dr. Johnson offers no context. And so I ask him, "Compared to what?"

The cost of untreated addiction is incalculable. From drunken driving injuries and deaths, crime, homelessness, visits to the emergency room, lost profits in the workplace, and the millions of broken lives of fractured families everywhere, nobody is immune to addiction's impact. There are scores of credible studies about how treatment reduces these problems.

Also, research and scientists tell us that such treatment is effective when compared to outcome data for other incurable, chronic illnesses like asthma, diabetes, and hypertension. Relapse is more common for those illnesses than for addiction.

I've never been a numbers guy. I leave that to the experts. And even though statistics never lie, experts on both sides of a contentious issue like this one can spin the numbers to support their cases. Instead, I prefer to tap into the experiences of the real experts who aren't in this debate: the addicts and alcoholics who gathered last Monday around a table at their meeting place on Summit Avenue in Saint Paul, Minnesota.

In that crowded room were people in recovery. A middle-aged mother who once had seven years of sobriety but now was back with seven days. A police officer with a sudden urge to drink a six-pack of beer even though he tasted his last cold one about fifteen years ago. A student from St. Thomas University who announced it was his twenty-first birthday and his twentieth month of sobriety on the same day. There was also a woman who nervously admitted it was the first time she'd even been to a Twelve Step meeting. She had been drinking the day before.

I was there, too, clean and sober and reasonably sensible since 1994 after multiple treatments.

There were no failures in that room, only varying degrees of success. Our own experiences highlight what works and what doesn't. Those experiences are what got us to that place in the beginning and what keep us coming back there day after month after year.

My column got plenty of attention, most of it positive. As they say in the Twelve Step program, "Take what works and leave the rest."

But don't just take it from me. As I mentioned, I am not objective.

Dr. Ronald Earl Smith, a U.S. Navy captain who has spent the past thirty-three years treating alcoholism in the military, said it best in his pointed response to Dr. Johnson: "Two million sober members of AA . . . will see his [claim] and know how wrong he is for them."

We'll explore more about what Twelve Step meetings can offer people coming out of treatment in chapter 5.

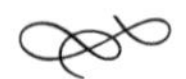

CHAPTER 5

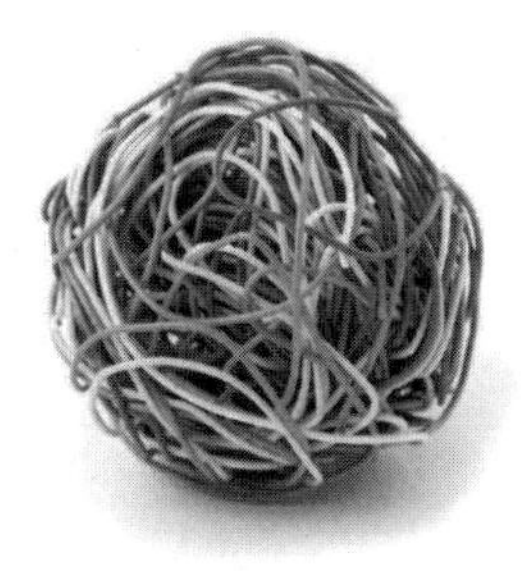

Peer Recovery: From "I" to "We"

At the apex of the battle of Antietam in September 1862, a desperate soldier cast his eyes to the heavens, certain the bloodiest single day of the American Civil War could never end.

"The sun slides backwards across the sky and night won't come," he wrote. But the night did come, just as night always ends each day. Somehow he survived his eternal day on the battlefield. Thousands of his friends and foes did not.

Suddenly your fight will be over too. You'll be on the other side of that last drink or drug. It took years to quit, years of stopping and starting and pledges and promises. All sorts of travails had people chasing after you and you chasing after something you sensed was within reach but couldn't grab on to, running like sand through your fingers.

Now picture it: it is the next day, the day after that long night finally came. Perhaps this day arrives when you wake up in a dirty jail cell, covered in your own vomit. Or in a hospital room, hazily grasping at memories to figure out what happened and who else you harmed. Or within the unfamiliar surroundings of a treatment facility. Or at home in bed, your skull splitting with a wicked hangover and your guts feeling as though they're about to burst out of your belly.

Wherever you are, you've somehow put yesterday behind you, even as your body still cries out, "Soothe me. Just go back for one more. For a moment. That's all. Right now." You snap to attention, all your energy, what's left of it, focused on where to find something, anything, to suture the gaping wounds—physical, mental, emotional wounds, all oozing like an infection. Then you're jolted by the futility of it all; you're tired, beaten up, and beaten down—but not beaten to death. It's over. It really is over this time. You've stopped.

And when you've stopped, the blinding blur of all those days running together abruptly ceases, and it is the next day. The day when you know the pursuit of oblivion isn't worth the terrible toll on you or the people around you. The day you grab on to something that feels different this time. The day you start to get well by putting behind you the substances that came so close to destroying you.

A lot of us are out here on the other side of yesterday. You'll start meeting some of us if you go through a treatment program. And an even larger community of people have crossed to the other side in the thousands of Twelve Step peer-recovery meetings going on every day.

A COMMUNITY OF "WE"

Most treatment centers will encourage their clients to join a Twelve Step support group when they finish treatment. Some, especially outpatient programs, make going to meetings a requirement, even if they don't focus on the Twelve Steps in their approach to treatment. They do this because these meetings are free, they are usually readily available (especially Alcoholics Anonymous and Narcotics Anonymous), and millions of people find that regularly attending these groups and applying the Twelve Step program of recovery in their daily lives keep them sober and drug-free. For alcoholics and many addicts as well, if they were actively using both alcohol and other drugs, AA is the program of choice. NA is favored by others whose drug of choice was heroin or another street drug. Of course, some people prefer NA just because of the mix of people and their different take on the Twelve Steps.

One of the great benefits of peer recovery, no matter which meetings you go to, is the sense of community. Community is especially important for addicts whose isolation and loneliness have been hallmarks of their disease. You'll hear a lot of people say that this is the first place in a long time where they felt as though they belonged. They have changed their "I" to "we."

SHARING OUR STORIES

In World War II, Colonel Lewis Melvin "Mel" Schulstad flew forty-four combat missions as the commanding pilot of a Boeing B-17, even though he could have gone home after twenty-five and the average survival rate of a bomber crew was about five missions. He always marveled that he made it through the war, and not just because for two years the enemy was trying to kill him every day. It turns out another foe just as lethal as the Nazis but a bit more subtle was stalking him too: alcohol.

For twenty more years after World War II ended, alcohol waged another war on Colonel Schulstad. Then one day in 1965, an incident involving top secret documents, a blackout, and a hangover in a hotel near the Pentagon finally convinced him it was time to stop.

He recounted his story to me in one of our visits:

> I called the Army chaplain and said, "I am here. I am a full colonel. I am very drunk, I am very sick, I've got lots of trouble, and I need help."

The chaplain put him in touch with a couple of strangers who were very different from him in so many ways, but they were fundamentally like him in one very important way—they, too, were alcoholics. They had found the answer to their problem and were willing to help him with his, starting by telling him their stories.

> "For the first time in my life I realized I wasn't alone," he said. "I'd known plenty of other alcoholics—

> hell, that was my crowd. But I didn't know any who'd stopped drinking and recovered until these men opened their lives to me. From them it hit me, "Well, what do you know, I'm not unique after all."

Not long before he died in 2012 at age ninety-three, I visited Mel at his bedside to say good-bye. His eyes remained closed during the hour we were together. It was difficult for him to talk. His sentences were short and his voice was shaky.

"Why," I asked him, "why did we make it? Why did we stop pursuing oblivion, get help, pull our lives together, and find recovery when so many others hadn't? Why did we survive?"

There was a long pause. Mel knew the answer. He had to summon the strength to articulate it, and then only in a bare whisper.

"God saw us through it all so we could tell others our stories." And what a story Mel had to tell.

Part of his story forms a thread in the resilient fabric of what we've come to know and admire as the "greatest generation." Mel was one of millions of Americans born and reared during the Great Depression who came of age in World War II. Their collective experiences and accomplishments poured into our consciousness through the work of journalists like Studs Terkel, Stephen Ambrose, and Tom Brokaw, inspiring us with their courage and willingness to put their lives on the line for our shared values. Another important part of Mel's story, his struggle with and recovery from alcoholism, makes him a member of what I'm calling the "we generation," people who were no longer destined to follow the path that for centuries had doomed so many others to a life of destitution, despair, crime, and ultimately, insanity and death.

Sparked by the advent of the Twelve Step movement beginning in the 1930s, the proliferation of peer-led self-help groups had a lot to do with these stories of experience, strength, and hope offering a forum for proving that help was possible.

AA had its real start in 1935 with Bill Wilson telling Dr. Bob Smith his story—his history of out-of-control drinking, hitting bottom in a hospital where he had a spiritual awakening that led to him stop drinking, and discovering what his new life was like without alcohol, including the realization that he needed to help other alcoholics to stay sober himself. Stories are so important to the AA program that the first chapter of *Alcoholics Anonymous,* the textbook for that program, opens with Bill Wilson's story. Not only that, the second half of the book consists of a wide range of people's stories of recovery, told using Bill's original model: telling what it was like, what happened, and what it's like now. Hearing the stories of people like us, as much as learning the science of addiction, shows us not only that addiction is an illness but that there's something we can do about it.

For many of us, though, this doesn't happen right away.

A memory from junior high school: Some guy, who seemed to me to be crusty and old with nothing to say relevant to my life, visited my Health and Wellness class to tell his story of drinking and recovery, in AA lovingly called a "drunk-a-log." And although the details faded long ago, I do recall that his tale made no sense to me, because I wasn't ready to see that he was talking about me as well as himself.

The same thing happened in college: There was a campus lecture, sparsely attended, that I covered as a reporter for the school paper. By this juncture, my pursuit of oblivion was picking up speed. I felt itchy on the inside about what the speakers shared outside, but they seemed a lot worse than me, so I dismissed their stories of loss of control and descent into the hell of addiction as something I would surely avoid.

Only a decade later, when I was locked in the psych ward with another odd lot of people I'd never met, did I begin to really grasp the futility that cast us together. We were like shipwreck survivors adrift in an overcrowded lifeboat—a couple of black women without teeth who looked forty years beyond their ages, a guy hooked up to an IV in the final stages of AIDS, a young Hispanic mother who barely spoke English, and a well-heeled, formerly successful white guy from the sheltered 'burbs in a selfish love affair with crack cocaine. That last guy was me. Those of us in the group were different in every way except one, the reason we were there. We wanted to stop getting drunk or stoned all the time. We wanted to live.

Those first meetings weren't voluntary. As temporary residents of the ward, we had no choice except to be there. But in our circle conversations, storytelling always dominated, precipitated by the obvious questions, "Who are you and why are you here?" All at once, each of us became a new student in a room full of instructors and an experienced instructor in a room filled with students. We had as much to learn as to teach. Whether delivered with academic eloquence or punctuated with expletives, the language we spoke resonated, because what we shared was essentially the same. What counted was hearing and telling stories that proved to be the catalyst to hear, see, and know the possibility of change.

One of the great contributions of peer-recovery meetings like those in AA and NA is that they give alcoholics and addicts a time and a place to congregate, sometimes daily or weekly, but most importantly, on a regular basis, to swap stories of our experiences. It doesn't matter whether we are two days out of the psych ward or three decades past our last high: our stories keep us coming back to talk or just to listen, to laugh and cry, to offer empathy or find solace, to tap resolve or affirm a truth. Always there is something to learn, to take away until next time.

PEER-RECOVERY MEETINGS

You'll find meetings in most communities, with a wide selection available in metropolitan areas. Meetings happen everywhere—in treatment facilities, jails, church basements, coffee shops, and community centers. There are even impromptu meetings on cruise ships, in airports, and on vacation tours, usually heralded over the loudspeaker or by handwritten signs using the code phrase "Friends of Bill W."

The best way to find meetings is to get a recommendation from your counselor if you're in treatment or from someone you know and trust who goes to AA or NA. You can also find a number for the AA or NA in your community by looking in the phone book or searching the Internet. The websites for AA (www.aa.org) and for NA World Services (www.na.org) have meeting finders you can use to search out meetings in your area.

COMMON TYPES OF PEER-RECOVERY MEETINGS

Here's a quick guide to the most common kinds of meetings available:

Open meetings

This refers to the fact that people who don't self-identify as alcoholics may attend the meetings. Many of the Speaker meetings (see below) are open meetings. Open meetings are usually clearly marked on websites or in literature announcing them.

Closed meetings

Only people who recognize they are alcoholics and have a sincere desire to stop drinking may attend these meetings. Most of the Step meetings, for example, are closed meetings. Again, such meetings are usually clearly marked online and in printed material.

Speaker meetings

These meetings feature a speaker, either a volunteer from within the group or a guest from another group. The speakers usually tell their personal stories, but sometimes they'll speak to AA members about, for example, one of the Steps or a theme from the Big Book, *Alcoholics Anonymous.* These tend to be larger meetings, which may split into smaller groups following the speaker's talk.

Big Book meetings

As you would expect, these meetings focus very strongly on reading selections from the Big Book, followed by group discussion, which is usually focused on that topic.

Step meetings

My home group was a Step meeting and each week a member would volunteer to give a short talk regarding a Step (or a Tradition), which we would then discuss.

Topic meetings

A group member might want to discuss a certain topic relevant to AA members; for example, sponsorship or emotional sobriety. If other members agreed, that member would lead the meeting with a talk, usually relating that topic to the person's own experience.

Story meetings

In my old group, the sequence of running through the Steps could be put on hold for a week if a group member wanted the time to tell his or her story to the group. This is also what we did when we would do service work; for example, holding meetings at the county jail with inmates who wanted to learn about AA.

Combined group meetings

There are occasions when two AA groups, with perhaps a mutual member or two, agree to merge meetings for a week to give everyone exposure to new people and fresh ideas.

Gender- or cultural-specific meetings

At first, this type of group may seem antithetical to the AA principle that the only requirement needed to attend a meeting is a desire to stop drinking. Sometimes for certain populations, though, special issues around staying sober have inspired them to create meetings that are either explicitly or implicitly limited by race or culture (African, Asian, or Native American groups), gender (men's and women's groups), sexual orientation (GLBT groups), or language (groups of recent Hispanic, Asian, or African immigrants). These groups are usually only found in larger cities where there are concentrations of people in these specific populations.

Some members with mental health or other special issues have formed separate organizations—for example, Double Trouble in Recovery and Dual Recovery Anonymous—to allow them to address their emotional and psychiatric problems along with their sobriety.

The first time you walk into a meeting, you probably won't know anyone, but then again, you may be surprised to run into someone you know and to see the person in a completely new light. I recall taking a dear friend to his first recovery meeting where he and his personal physician bumped into each other. "You?" each telegraphed to the other through surprised looks. Some people don't want anyone to recognize them and will drive a long way to avoid running into friends, family, or work associates, especially in smaller communities. For many of us, though, our sobriety is girded by the comfort of having fellow travelers in our community who see us on the street or in a store or at church.

Wherever you go, it's best to keep going to that same group at the same place at the same time each week. Give a group a chance; a lot of us are uncomfortable in the beginning, but if we give it time and get to know the people, we begin to feel the support from the "experience, strength, and hope" that can fill these rooms. And if you like the format and the people there, you can start calling it your "home group" and make that your default meeting.

On the other hand, if you've given a meeting a fair chance but you're still uncomfortable and don't feel this is the right group for you, then try other meetings. Whether it's the format or simply group chemistry, some meetings are more helpful than others, depending on your individual needs.

SPONSORS

As soon as possible, you should think about getting a sponsor. Hamilton B., in his book *Twelve Step Sponsorship,* defines a sponsor this way:

> A sponsor is someone who has been where we want to go in our Twelve Step program and knows something about how we can get there. His or her primary responsibility is to help us work the Twelve Steps by applying their principles to our lives.

He tells us the best way to find the right sponsor is to go to meetings and identify someone who is several years sober and drug-free and has things to say that you like, someone you identify with and trust. You can also ask recovering friends or other group members for suggestions. A sponsor should be the same gender you are; that is, unless you are gay or lesbian, in which case the opposite is true.

PARTICIPATION MYTHS

"I was an introvert before I ever started drinking, an introvert when I was drunk, and much later in treatment, the same," recalls Lynne G., the owner of a thriving bakery in Northern California. "It was even worse *after* I stopped drinking. . . . Sitting in a room with a group of people I didn't know, well, it terrified me to no end." Her small town offered only a few Twelve Step meetings a week. She made herself go. A year later she's still hanging with the same group "and I'm still an introvert, except when I'm there."

A myth about Twelve Step meetings is that you're required to participate or otherwise engage in the discussion. Not true, except at the beginning, when people usually introduce themselves with their first names and their reasons for being there; for example, "My name is William; I'm an alcoholic and addict." Other than that, you don't have to say or do anything. I've heard reluctant newcomers give their name and nothing else, because they're not yet sure what their problem is or aren't comfortable with the label. In meetings at which members share for a few minutes, it is okay to pass, too. And when the basket or hat is passed around for donations, generally a buck or two, you can pass on that as well—there are no dues or other financial obligations.

Another myth is that Twelve Step meetings are like group therapy and people will be analyzing you and telling you how to live your life. Actually there's a tradition in AA for "no cross talk." Usually, but only if they feel like it, every person shares his or her thoughts on that meeting's topic, which is often one of the Twelve Steps, or a person may say a few words about how the previous week has gone and then passes to the next person—and that's it. At Speaker meetings, most of the meeting is taken up with someone telling his or her story.

THE POWER OF "WE"

At one time, except for detox programs in hospitals and exclusive retreats where wealthy people went to dry out in a spa-like environment, Twelve Step meetings were all that was available for getting sober and drug-free. Then treatment programs based on the Minnesota Twelve Step Model began to emerge in the 1950s, and they eventually became a major portal for people through AA, NA, and other Twelve Step peer-recovery programs. Today a vast majority of us attend meetings to stay in recovery or to regain it after a slip of a few days or a full-blown relapse lasting years. Still, Twelve Step meetings are a lifeline for millions of people, whether they're coming out of treatment, drug court, or a physician's office. For every first-time "newbie," there's an old-timer, and for every slipper or slider, there's a rock-solid veteran to offer a path from powerlessness to accountability, resentment to gratitude.

Alcoholics Anonymous Twelve Step programs work exactly for these reasons. But it isn't for everyone. Many people stop using through churches, alternative recovery-oriented groups, and group therapy facilitated by a counselor. Many such approaches offer the intimacy of regular conversation and themes that stress honest introspection and self-improvement. In these groups, too, the power of persuasion and conviction usually lies in personal testimonials. Stories of hopeless desperation under the influence, followed by that moment of clarity, and the conviction of the possibilities of redemption, are what bring us together to find strength and healing through a power greater than self, the power of "we."

RECOVERY AND THE TWELVE STEPS

In March 2012, a groundbreaking national survey by the Partnership at DrugFree.Org and the New York State Office of Alcoholism and Substance Abuse Services asked 2,526 adults this question: "Did you once have a problem with drugs or alcohol, but no longer do?" According to the survey data, one in ten respondents said yes, which the survey correlates to about 23 million of us in the United States who don't have that endless run of bad days under the influence anymore. The survey called the answer "one simple way of describing recovery from drug and alcohol abuse or addiction."

A very "simple way," indeed, because there may be truth to the saying "a drug is a drug is a drug," but people who use these substances view their "problem," and also view their search for a solution, very differently. My sense is that the only real takeaway from the survey is that a lot of us are pretty certain we're better now.

A PLACE OF RECOVERY

What does this mean, exactly, to be better or, as the survey describes it, to be in a place of "recovery"? What does this place look like? How does it feel? What are the implications?

Through the years, my own informal, unscientific, and certainly flawed queries of people who had the problem elicit responses like these about what it is like for them since their old days under the influence:

"I don't get high anymore; that's about it."

"Finally I have real, live hope."

"I'm free."

"Today I am clean and sober, just for today."

"My family respects me finally."

"The cravings are gone."

"The cops don't scare me anymore, because I'm straight and doing nothing wrong."

"I got back my dignity."

"God found me . . . no, I found God."

"It's all ancient history. I don't think about that part of my life anymore and I'm glad for it."

There's seldom a pessimistic chord among us, we who have put the problem behind us in one way or another. In this body politic is a good number, close to a majority perhaps, who do use the noun "recovery" to describe themselves and where they are right now, on that other side of yesterday. People have reclaimed what they lost or have come to experience something new as a direct result of what they've gained by changing their lives.

RECOVERY TERMINOLOGY

"I am in recovery." You hear it all the time in Twelve Step meetings. Not just as a noun either, but as an adjective, as in "I am a recovering alcoholic" to describe an ongoing process that many people believe is essential to avoid falling back into the clutches of alcohol or other drugs.

To stay "recovered," all you need to do is never forget how bad it was before you ever uttered that word.

A couple of pioneers back me on this too, I think. Bill Wilson, who was the co-founder of AA with Dr. Bob Smith, and Marty Mann, who was the first woman to achieve long-term recovery in AA, both advocated for use of the term *recovered.* Consider this excerpt from *A Biography of Mrs. Marty Mann,* chronicling the life of this vocal public advocate for treatment of alcoholism:

> Marty also felt strongly that AAs should refer to themselves as *recovered,* not *recovering.* Bill Wilson firmly advocated the use of *recovered,* too. For these two pioneers, *recovered* meant "I'm well today"—*recovering* meant "I'm still sick." [emphasis added]

In 2004, Faces & Voices of Recovery (www.facesandvoices ofrecovery.org) commissioned a "first of its kind" survey on how everyone besides addicts viewed recovery and concluded "the public does not know what *recovery* means." When asked their definition of somebody in recovery, 62 percent said it meant the person is "trying to stop using alcohol or illicit drugs." Only 22 percent said it meant the person had actually stopped. And get this: according to the survey, "even those who know someone in recovery overwhelmingly (62 percent) believe that someone in recovery is '*trying* to stop using alcohol or drugs.'"

The nomenclature of recovery bamboozles policy makers, dumbs down debate in the media, confuses public perception, and divides the professionals whose jobs are to help people with this problem. It obscures the truth about what works and what doesn't. The lack of benchmarks to measure progress in recovery, set goals, and achieve success continues to foster misperceptions about addiction, about treatment for those who need it, and about recovery for those who want it.

WORKING THE TWELVE STEPS—OR NOT

Even within the ranks of the largest community of people who seek to avoid the ravages of addiction, those who ascribe to the Twelve Steps, there often exists a "one size fits all" doctrinaire attitude that flies in the face of the illness's chronic dynamic. If you are not continuously "clean and sober," as it goes, then you are not "in recovery." If you are not "working the Steps," as they say, you are not "in recovery," even though you may be abstinent. In both instances, nothing is further from the truth.

I know hundreds of people whose sobriety is interrupted by episodic use of the substances, what some clinicians call "lapses," but whose aspirations for recovery never cease. Many others I know once sought help in the Twelve Steps, stuck with the program for a while, got what they needed, and then stopped following that program. They are still drug-free. There are those who count themselves in recovery assisted by medications, such as methadone and buprenorphine, or doctor-prescribed medications, such as Xanax or other drugs, to manage anxiety and other mental illnesses, and they no longer turn to alcohol or street drugs to medicate their illnesses. Certainly among people in the survey who "once [had] a problem with drugs or alcohol, but no longer do," there are many who simply leave well enough alone, put their drug use in the past, and find what they need by making life full in other ways, such as attending church, practicing yoga, running marathons, doing meditation, traveling to the Seven Wonders of the World, pursuing a career, parenting, or donating their time as a volunteer contributing to a cause in which they believe. It's likely that these people are finding in these activities that same "power greater than self" that others have found going to meetings and working the Twelve Steps.

It is neither my place nor my intention to discount any pathway to a healthier life without substances as long as it begins with this conscious notion of being "recovered." If we keep front and center this perspective that alcohol and other drugs caused us never-ending problems and that we can no longer control their use, then we always have a jumping-off point from which to move forward, whether it is the day after yesterday or decades from now. What matters is that we never forget how bad things were when those substances ruled our lives, despite our best intentions.

I'd like to now focus on what being in recovery is all about for me and for so many of us who believe there is much more to overcoming addiction than simply stopping. For millions of us, the crisis of the moment that gets us to stop evolves into a lifelong commitment to facing and dealing with what happens after we've stopped. In this way, addiction is like diabetes, hypertension, and other chronic illnesses, including cancer, that must be managed day to day over a lifetime. Experts call it "disease management," and it applies to alcoholism and drug addiction, although for our purposes, I prefer to label it "recovery management," because it sounds more optimistic and empowering. Also, recovering from addiction involves not only nurturing the body and mind but the spirit as well, and as you'll see, one of the most effective ways to nurture the spirit is by making a commitment to help "our fellow travelers" who are still suffering. They are as important to us as we are to them.

One of my mentors in recovery, Paul L.—a combat veteran of World War II, a newspaperman, and the father of two sons, whose drinking jeopardized everything—put it best: "In 1961 I sought treatment, desperate to change what booze was doing to my life. What I ended up getting for that effort was an entirely changed life." He died in 2006, having never taken a drink again. In those years, he helped many others change their lives as well. People like me.

DESIGN FOR LIVING

What made that life change possible for Paul L. was the design for living that also works for people like me and millions of others who call themselves recovering alcoholics and addicts, people who have vowed not to return to the clutches of addiction. I'm talking about the prescription for recovery that has changed nary a word since it was published in 1939 in the Big Book of Alcoholics Anonymous and summed up in the Twelve Steps (see appendix E for the full text; see also appendix F for the NA Twelve Steps).

These Twelve Steps are a program of action that empowers people with the chronic illness of addiction to actively engage in the solution of a healthier life. Such action and change never happens perfectly; nobody with a chronic illness gets well and stays well without slips and slides back into the mud hole, the messy behaviors that are as much about our humanness as our illness. In my own recovery I've been there myself, more than once through the years. But the Twelve Step program empowers you within a framework that recognizes the unique physical, emotional, and mental characteristics of addiction, the importance of putting down the substance once and for all, and the long-term value of "an entirely changed life," as Paul L. so simply put it. The process is measured in day-to-day effort and tallied as years or decades of progress.

Scores of books have been written about why and how these Steps work—or don't. My "It Works" column in chapter 4 has let you know my stance on *whether* it works, so we won't rehash that argument. (And you can visit appendix A for further reading ideas.) We just need to understand why these

Twelve Steps—more than any other method or program—have been a successful path to recovery for so many people. Learning about the Twelve Steps might help you understand why this path might work for you or somebody you love. So let's take a look at exactly what those Steps say.

ONE ADDICT'S TAKE ON THE TWELVE STEPS

If you decide to go into a treatment program that incorporates these Steps in its treatment plan, and certainly if you go to AA or NA, you'll get a lot of different perspectives on each Step to deepen your understanding and make them your own. As a brief introduction for you, here are some things I've picked up from other recovering people in regard to the Twelve Steps.

Sanity

With the first three Steps, we face the fact that we have a disease, that we need help to get better, and we decide to do what's necessary to get that help.

STEP ONE

> We admitted we were powerless over alcohol—that our lives had become unmanageable.

The most important word in this First Step is also the most important word in the recovery process: *we*. Remember, addiction is an illness of isolation, loneliness, and shame. The antidote to it starts when we embrace that we don't have to be alone anymore, and in fact, we shouldn't if we really want to improve our prospects for recovery. What a relief to find others who understand our predicament, share our experiences, and aspire to the same outcome. It's even more inspiring to discover that "we" may include people from all walks of life, and of both genders, and all ages, cultures, and beliefs. These are people who can be as different from us as people in any random gathering—except for the common denominator that we suffer from the same illness and have the same desire to stop drinking and drugging.

What about this notion of being *powerless?* Don't we pride ourselves on having as much willpower as the next person? But where alcohol and other drugs are concerned, by the time somebody has told us to read this Step, we know deep down what *powerlessness* means. Haven't we tried repeatedly to control or stop our drinking and to mitigate the consequences on our own and with all our willpower offers us—and failed? And with that failure, we know all too well how we lose the ability to manage most other aspects of our lives. We're not that different from diabetics or people with cancer who may have all the will in the world, too, to beat their illness. But like us, they need professional help and the support of others; they can't do it on their own.

Yet powerlessness isn't an excuse for our bad behavior, for the havoc we created when we were using. Remember, we're not responsible for having the illness, but we are responsible for doing what it takes to recover. Accepting our powerlessness actually empowers us to stop being part of the problem and to start working toward the solution.

STEP TWO

Came to believe that a Power greater than ourselves could restore us to sanity.

Just as the progression of the illness of addiction is a process that doesn't happen overnight, with this Step we get our first inkling that the solution to it is equally an evolving process. "Came to believe" doesn't mean we get it all at once. Usually our awareness unfolds as we stumble along, get up, and stumble again, consciously reaching a point at which we do acknowledge that there's got to be something bigger and more powerful than our own intense desire to drink and use despite the harmful consequences. This is the "insanity" we experience when we continue to try again and again something that hasn't worked and to expect different results. So what is this Power that can restore our sanity? It depends. But now we've reached a point that we know the Power isn't us on our own, and we at least believe there is something else out there.

STEP THREE

Made a decision to turn our will and our lives over to the care of God *as we understood Him.*

Here's one of those "Now what?" moments that can be like a pie in the face or a lightning bolt from the sky or a whisper in the ear, depending on your perspective. What I hope is that it will be a moment of clarity that finally speaks to you with a simple truth: I can't and don't want to do this on my own anymore.

At this moment we don't give up. We give in. We begin to ask for help. We start to accept help. Finally, we are open to the prospect that there is another way. This is where our will—call it call *willpower* if you want—counts for something, because we become willing to change. We are ready to apply ourselves to the process that leads to a solution.

I know, some of you are scared off by the word *God.* This is usually the point at which some critics shake their fingers and say, "There, you see, it's a cult that's trying to push religions down our throats." Certainly God is all over the Twelve Steps. The original authors labeled this Power as God because that's what they understood it to be from their own experiences in a Judeo-Christian culture. But they also had the wisdom to use the terms *Higher Power* and *Power greater than ourselves,* knowing that many alcoholics and addicts are from religious traditions that don't use the term *God* as their deity, not to mention the many who are agnostics or even atheists. Many people who have struggled with the term *God* treat it as an acronym for "Good, Orderly, Direction." Others treat the Twelve Step program itself and their AA or NA group conscience as their Higher Power. For others, their Power is nature. People who are really ready to give the Steps a try have found many creative and meaningful ways to conceive of a Power greater than themselves that represents a healing force more powerful than their craving for alcohol or other drugs.

Whew! The first three Steps, bang, bang, bang! But as you probably can tell, when you really let these ideas sink in, following these Steps is not that easy. Internalizing these Steps and making them real in our lives can take a while.

Often people will reach the First Step painfully aware that they have a problem, only to lose their grip and continue their plunge downward. You can make it to the Second Step and the same thing can happen. The false promises of the high, the delusion that this time it will be different, can sweep you away. Finally you may come back to that place where you're so desperate that you grab and hold on to the promise in the Second Step and are ready to make the decision asked of you in Third Step.

For some, though, it happens in a flash; suddenly the other side of yesterday is now and you are ready to try and "recover" what you've lost, pick up the pieces, and put back together a broken life. It takes a lot of work. It is an inside job and an outside job, because we've not only wounded ourselves but caused all of that collateral damage we talked about in earlier chapters.

Such collateral damage is one thing that sets addiction apart from other illnesses. You've probably noticed I compare addiction to other chronic illnesses in my writing and when I'm speaking on behalf of Hazelden in my public advocacy work. I do get a fair amount of criticism from people when I invoke addiction in the same breath as diabetes, heart disease, or cancer, especially from people who suffer from those complicated illnesses.

"You addicts asked for your problems, your 'illness,' and you deserve what you get! I've got diabetes and I've survived skin cancer and I didn't ask for or deserve either," said a woman who angrily confronted me in the middle of a speech.

She's right in that we are responsible for taking the first drink or hit. And once we know this is an illness, we are responsible for doing what it takes to get better. And she's right that there are differences in our illnesses, but I see us alcoholics and addicts as needing to take our recovery process beyond taking a medicine like insulin or eating more healthfully. We must move beyond recognition and realization to being accountable for our illness, which we'll consider in the next six Steps.

Accountability: Steps Four through Nine

Most of us now understand that our drinking or drugging is a symptom of a bigger problem that is as much at the root of addiction as is the brain's wiring and the body's physical reaction to mood-altering chemicals. We have been battling the shame of our addiction and our own human imperfections for too long. We've tried to bury these feelings where nobody else can find them. We've known they are there, even if we can't label them. We've carried shame and resentments around and pursued oblivion to avoid facing these feelings, bouncing back and forth between believing that we're not deserving of love and respect and believing we never get enough and deserve more. By holding these delusional beliefs and repressed feelings, we added fuel to the fire, resulting in irrational behaviors that harmed other people. Here is where we bring to bear our full accountability to recover from our illness, and it takes hard work over a long time.

STEP FOUR

Made a searching and fearless moral inventory of ourselves.

STEP FIVE

Admitted to God, to ourselves, and to another human being the exact nature of our wrongs.

STEP SIX

Were entirely ready to have God remove all these defects of character.

STEP SEVEN

Humbly asked Him to remove our shortcomings.

STEP EIGHT

Made a list of all persons we had harmed, and became willing to make amends to them all.

STEP NINE

Made direct amends to such people wherever possible, except when to do so would injure them or others.

There's plenty to deal with in the accountability Steps. It takes a lot of time, too, to clean up our messes, time that requires we be free from the substances we had used to mask, suppress, or medicate these feelings. Only when we stop getting high or drunk do we begin to accurately and completely come to terms with this important part of our illness. Taking stock with the Fourth Step lays it all out. And by facing our character flaws and the harms we've done, we discover our real strengths and that we are basically good but flawed humans.

When we've uncovered in the Fourth Step the resentments and flaws that made us restless, irritable, and discontented in the first place, we need to let go of them, initially in the Fifth Step by telling another person what we've uncovered—both the flaws and the strengths—and then by turning everything in our inventory over to our Higher Power with Steps Six and Seven. They've all got to go if we want to get and stay healthy. No pill, no prison sentence, no wave of a magic wand is going to do it for us. We've got to want to change, and to change means firmly walking the ground these six Steps cover. Recognition. Responsibility. Redemption.

I could never stay recovered until I plunged into this process headfirst and dove deeply into who I really was inside. I had tried this before, but I had never exactly followed the recipe, mostly because I was afraid of what I would find and, worse, afraid to tell anyone what I had found. The result was predictable. Eventually I started drinking and drugging again in vain attempts to keep secretly at bay what I wouldn't let go of. I was like a long-distance runner who complains of blisters, but won't empty his shoes of the stones that cause the sores. At least, that's how I was until the day I stopped.

I vividly recall laying myself open in a one-on-one conversation with one of my wiser mentors, Bob. C., a fellow journalist at CNN, where I was working when I relapsed in 1994. That day I told him everything about myself, even the two or three secrets I had sworn I would never reveal to anyone. When I did, he leaned back in his chair and said, "You too, huh?" And in that instant I realized I wasn't alone in the shame and regret that is so much a force of my illness. By telling somebody else, I spoke this truth to myself, too, and what I heard myself say made it easier to accept who I was and how I wanted to change. I stopped running.

If uncovering and admitting the truth to ourselves is so important in Step One, why are the "God Steps" of Five through Seven vital too? Because by now we understand the role a Higher Power plays in helping us see ourselves, share ourselves, and change ourselves. If we've come this far, we know what's possible with the surrender that comes with faith in the program and in a Power greater than ourselves: a life free from substances. Faith that you don't have to do it all alone.

And that brings us to Steps Eight and Nine.

No alcoholic or addict is free from the regret of hurting others, especially our family and friends. Our Step Eight list of the people we've harmed can feel like a ball and chain. To free ourselves, we must first recognize that not all of the harm came when we were drunk or stoned, but also in those behaviors and actions that came out of our illness—behaviors born of our selfishness, dishonesty, resentment, and fear.

So in Step Nine we apologize. We make restitution. We ask for another chance. Our hope is to restore our ties and our integrity with people. But not all will be necessarily forgiven, now or perhaps ever. Some relations have been forever altered and others have been mortally harmed. We may be forced to grieve what we've lost and cannot retrieve. That's why the motivation for making amends is really about owning our absolute responsibility for the harm we caused, without mitigation.

Again, this gives us the clarity to come to terms with the totality of our illness. Whether others forgive us or not, we can only forgive ourselves. If we can't, we risk living a life intoxicated, if not with alcohol and other drugs, then with regret and resentment toward the people around us and, worst of all, toward ourselves.

Maintenance: Steps Ten through Twelve

The last three Steps of the Twelve Step recovery process are known as the maintenance Steps. They serve as the daily touchstones so vital to staying healthy through the distractions and temptations of our busy, unpredictable lives.

STEP TEN

> Continued to take personal inventory and when we were wrong promptly admitted it.

"Wait a minute," you may be wondering. "Didn't you just describe that arduous process?"

Yes, mostly. We clean the messes we caused in our addiction. But guess what? We're still human! Our motives aren't always pure. We make mistakes and do things in recovery that everybody else does at one time or another, except for us such missteps and motives are inherently risky in the same way that a snowball rolling down a hill can pick up mass and speed and become an ominous avalanche. If you stop the snowball before it gets going, it stays little and doesn't become a big deal. We're the same way. Even after we've cleaned house, we do things we know are wrong or against the recovery principles we strive to live by. When something like that happens, we identify it, accept it, and correct it before it gets very far.

Once I was rushing through Chicago's O'Hare airport to make a connecting flight home. My addiction to the *New*

York Times unmet, I stopped at a newsstand to grab a fix. The line to the cashier was too long; I'd never get on the plane if I waited. So I rolled up the paper and ran to my gate without paying. It was "only" a buck, I rationalized. But after two minutes in my seat, I knew what I had done was wrong, because it was dishonest.

Now this had nothing directly to do with drinking or drugging because at that point I had been sober for a decade. But here's the point: in recovery we tend to notice the behaviors we masked, buried, or denied when we were using. Although dishonesty is unhealthy for anybody, for an addict, it's potentially deadly if it becomes that snowball that sets our character flaws and resentments in motion again. It bothered me like a stone in my shoe. My personal inventory, in which I'd identified dishonesty as one of my character flaws, caught me. The next time I was in the airport concourse, I handed the cashier a dollar. "For what?" she asked. "A newspaper I read two months ago," I answered, and I apologized. I am not sure she quite understood, but it didn't matter. I understood.

Of course, it is always a hell of a lot easier to promptly admit a mistake when it involves a purloined newspaper worth a buck rather than something more egregious. The whopper mistakes I've made over the years—and, living any length of time, we're all prone to make some—pose a bigger challenge. I've not always handled them exactly the same way. When I don't deal with a problem right away, it gets messier. When I do step up, own it, and try make it right, eventually it gets sorted out. I've had a lot of practice.

STEP ELEVEN

Sought through prayer and meditation to improve our conscious contact with God *as we understood Him,* praying only for knowledge of His will for us and the power to carry that out.

If life is a journey, not a destination, then making contact with and staying connected to your Higher Power is an odyssey. Fortunately, being a Buddhist monk, a celibate nun, a soothsayer, or a prophet like Moses isn't a prerequisite to take this trek. Anybody can do it, anywhere, anytime, any way you like, and it doesn't have to become your vocation either. But to maintain our fit spiritual condition, to continue to heal the spirit as well as the body and mind, we addicts have to do some version of this Step.

For me, I do this Step at least once a day to keep me grounded and aware of my priorities. On many days, the cacophony of life's incessant obligations and distractions make it difficult to "work the Steps," as people in the program say. It ain't that easy. Who's got the time or energy to apply this twelve-point recipe exactly the way it is written? Not me. Not always. But not an early morning passes or bedtime comes before I have deliberately sat still long enough (know that for me fifteen minutes is a long time) to connect to God as I understand God. I keep it simple. In the morning my "conscious contact" goes like this: "Thank you, God, for the gift of another day. Thank you for all the good things that have come my way as a result of how I choose to live my life." At night it goes like this: "Thank you, God, for the gift of another day. A good day or a bad day, but another day I lived sober."

When we connect to a Higher Power, we always discover gratitude—or at least the strength to endure whatever comes our way. "My worst day sober is better than my best day drunk," some people say, and they mean it, because no matter the circumstances, we don't have to be stoned or drunk anymore to face our problems, and that simple truth affirms that we can endure. When my twenty-year relationship ended with the mother of our three children, my grief was like a dark sky; it covered everything. I hung on, though, by flexing that spiritual muscle that kept me connected to my Higher Power. I knew I was never alone.

A few months ago, in discussing the Eleventh Step, I poked at this notion of seeking God's will. "I don't know what God's will is for me," I said. A wiser man among us, Rick, pushed back with something I'd never heard before. "William, I suspect you know more about what God's will is for you than what you're letting on." Later I realized he was right. If nothing else, I believe that God's will is about me putting forth my best effort to stay recovered.

STEP TWELVE

> Having had a spiritual awakening as the result of these steps, we tried to carry this message to alcoholics, and to practice these principles in all our affairs.

If we've made it this far, we're destined to know the following points:

- Our addiction should have destroyed us, but didn't.
- The alternative to drinking is much more than simply not drinking.
- We become better human beings because of the good choices we make and the directions we follow.
- We can't keep what we don't give away; helping others helps us.

For me at least, this is what a spiritual awakening is all about. These four maxims have become absolutes that connect my whole life, even though I spend a fair amount of my life doing stuff that isn't directly related to my addiction or my recovery from it. Like lying on the couch watching football games on the weekend, fishing for bass on the longest day of the summer in Wisconsin, talking to my cats when nobody else is listening, watching my daughter hit a homerun on her last at-bat in her last softball game of the season, or taking my boys on college tours.

Actually, now that I've written this, I realize it all happens precisely because I recovered and am continually recovering, and I am grateful for the whole package, for everything I've been through, the bad with the good. I'm not craving a high; I'm not dead drunk, or even just dead. Instead, like a lot of others, I've turned around my life by turning the adversity of my addiction into the opportunity to change my life for the better, guided by these Twelve Step principles. An AA friend of mine, Bill P., who struggled long and hard with his character flaws, once told me, "The principles are the opposite of our defects of character, and it is our character defects that keep popping up, keep us coming back to these principles." Like Bill P., I am far from perfect in my sobriety. Some of my biggest issues and challenges have come since I got sober. But that's what AA's Twelve Step program is for: imperfect people living in an imperfect world who want to keep recovering, despite it all.

If it seems we've spent a lot of space and words on this one path to recovery, it's because this path has proven to be the most universally successful for the most people, no matter where they came from or their drug of choice. It's what has worked for me when everything else failed. As Bill W., the author of *Alcoholics Anonymous,* said in introducing the Steps in chapter 5 of that book: "Half measures avail us nothing. We stood at the turning point."

If you are at that turning point, I invite you to consider these Steps as an essential guide, your GPS navigation system on your path to sanity and freedom.

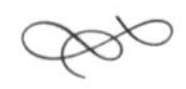

CHAPTER 6

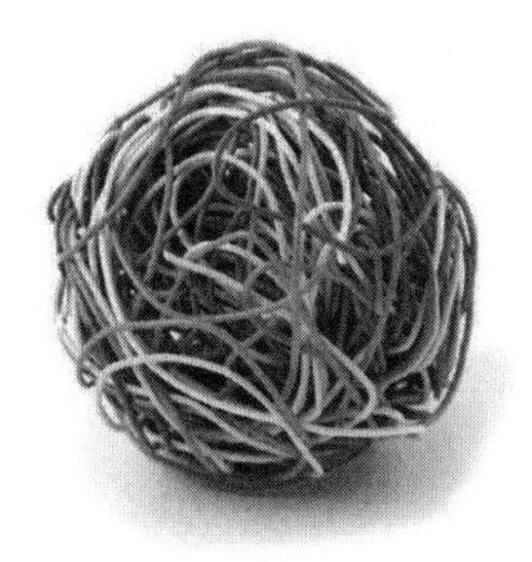

Relapse Isn't a Dirty Word

It is impossible to relapse if you've never tried to quit. You can't relapse if you don't think you should stop drinking and drugging in the first place. And if you construe recovery from addiction as something less than a starting point for complete abstinence, you can't relapse either. It's pretty simple: people "go back out" only after they've made a conscious, deliberate commitment to stop using. Sometimes relapse occurs as quickly as the day after. Decades can pass and still it can happen.

Relapse can occur with any chronic illness. Yet the label "relapse" is often associated with addiction to imply that somehow it is caused by the person's lack of will or moral failing. In other words, it's their fault that they started using again. Think about it: when a woman's breast cancer reappears, nobody says, "She's relapsed." When a man's coronary disease leads to another heart attack, we don't say, "He's at it again, relapsing." In those instances, it is the illness that returns, not the people returning to the illness.

That's not the prevailing view, though, when you or a loved one resumes using the substances that have caused everyone so much heartache. A friend of mine who has spent the past quarter century in and out of detox units, psych wards, high-priced treatment centers, and skid-row shelters said it best: "*Relapse* is a dirty word." No wonder the burden of shame weighs down many people who relapse to the point that their only escape seems to be to give in and give up.

It's a quirky paradox that for a chronic illness that cannot be cured, recovery from addiction is often only recognized and celebrated by the length of continuous abstinence. So when somebody takes a drink or a drug again, their tally of days, months, and years without drinking or using starts all over again from zero. It is interesting, too, that the competency of sponsors and other mentors in recovery is usually measured by how long they've gone without drinking or using, when some of the best lessons can be taught by those who have experienced a lapse and come back even more committed to staying sober and drug-free.

The fact is that we need to see relapse as part of the disease of addiction. That doesn't mean that recovery necessarily has to be interrupted by relapse. As important as it is to avoid relapse, though, it is just as important to understand that when relapse occurs, as it often does, you haven't really gone back to square one. There's no need to throw up your hands and give up altogether. For those of us who travel the route from addiction to redemption, this is a truth, if not a provable fact: most people who achieve lasting sobriety relapsed early on in their journey, and some do so many times before that last time when they finally say, "Enough is enough."

"Until we really believe we are powerless over the substance and certain that abstinence is the only way of life, we are just setting ourselves up for a relapse," said Mike S., thirty years into his own sobriety. "[When] people check the box, 'I am committed to remain sober, drinking or drugging again is nonnegotiable, and I am committed to following the recommendations of my counselors and sponsor,' then long-term sobriety becomes a reality."

A quick disclaimer: what follows isn't for people who seek to change their pattern of use but still choose to drink or drug. Plenty of people, having endured the ravages of substance abuse, choose to lead a healthier life and vow not to let their drinking and drugging get out of control again. But abstinence isn't one of their goals, so they find a way to cut down and use only occasionally, and sometimes they do just fine. Actually, these people wouldn't be diagnosed as alcoholics or addicts; instead they would fall under the classification of substance abusers. They aren't among that 8 to 10 percent of us who, because of the biological, psychological, and social factors in our makeup and personality, are unable to control our use once we start using.

We're using the term *relapse* to apply to people who recognize they have the disease of addiction, have decided to try to remain abstinent, but use mood- and mind-altering substances again. People like me. From the moment I entered treatment in 1989, I knew my problem was alcohol and other drugs, and I vowed to stop and was certain I would. Then I relapsed many times during the next five years. My last relapse, in 1994, combined with everything I had learned in treatment and in my stints in recovery, finally convinced me I could make it only if I worked hard to stop using and to stay stopped. Today, as much as I know about relapse, I feel like I'm still vulnerable to it happening again. The key for me, and an essential tool for anyone who wants to ward off the possibility of a relapse, is to never stop learning.

WHAT SPARKS RELAPSE?

Dr. William Silkworth, the doctor who treated Bill Wilson, the cofounder of Alcoholics Anonymous, identified the "phenomenon of craving" as a unique characteristic of the alcoholics he treated at his hospital in New York in the 1930s. Later on, MRIs and other advancements in technology allowed experts to see how the brains of alcoholics "lit up" not just under the direct influence of substances, but whenever images of liquor bottles and syringes and lines of cocaine were flashed before them. Some call it "euphoric recall," a steel trap set in the deepest recesses of memory or, as I like to put it, buried in a dark spot of the soul. That trap is primed to spring. If it does, we are once again caught in the excruciating grip of alcohol or other drugs. Always our pain is matched only by our utter bafflement of how it happened.

Twenty-four-year-old Lance S., an electrician, had been treated for alcoholism and managed to put together three months of recovery when he got picked up by the police on a warrant for unpaid traffic tickets. For a guy who had finally started the difficult process of turning his life around, it was an embarrassing, shame-filled moment, and he didn't know what to do. "I'd been in jail for three days, my wife was pissed and told me not to come home, the union boss didn't know where I'd been, and I had all of ten bucks in my pocket," he recalls. He was released from jail. On his way home in a cab, he passed his favorite bar and the urge for "one drink" took over. "Next thing I know I'm drunk. My wife is still pissed, the boss is still wondering where I am, and now I've got no money in my pocket and a $50 bar tab. So stunning, so sudden. I just don't know what happened."

Even people who are more established in recovery can step into the steel trap when they complacently believe they're safely past it and vigilance isn't paramount.

I know a lawyer in her forties who was treated and had been successful in sobriety for fifteen years. When she was on vacation in Mexico with her husband and two young children, her migraines sent her to a pharmacy where, to her surprise, she discovered she could purchase narcotics over the counter. "Never before had the idea even crossed my mind, but in a split second I convinced myself that Tylenol with codeine was a good idea for my migraines," she said. She stocked up before she came home and then used illegal Internet pharmacies to keep the supply flowing. "The first few times I was flooded with this uplifting relief from all of life's burdens. Of course, I knew better. . . . this was dangerous territory. It's just that once I started, I wanted more and more. I didn't want to stop, and then I knew I must. But couldn't." Within six months, she was a wreck. Her family was nearly destroyed. It took another treatment for her to get back on track. She's been drug-free again for seven years.

More than any other factor, it is this phenomenon of craving—sometimes dramatic and quick, sometimes coming on insidiously and slowly—that causes us to relapse. But why?

Science pins it on the mysterious intricacies of the addict's brain. Old-timers in Twelve Step recovery point to a failure to "follow the program." Critics of the concept of addiction as a disease say craving simply reflects a lack of willpower. Some religious people blame it on temptation by the devil. I think it comes down to this: the craving for another buzz overwhelms us and grows exponentially when we don't maintain a healthy respect for our disease and give in to the power of the delusion that we can drink and use like normal people. Combine this with our selective memory of the pleasure of the high, this "euphoric recall" blocks out all the havoc our drinking and drugging wreaks when it inevitably gets out of control, and you have the formula for relapse. Time may heal all wounds. But if we don't keep our mind on our inability to control our use after we take that first drink or hit, don't keep that knowledge foremost in our consciousness, no amount of time will serve as a seawall against the incessant tides of addiction.

That's not to suggest that years of sobriety don't improve our prospects of staying sober. Studies have shown that the longer we are substance-free, the less likely we are to step on the steel trap again, or to be washed out to sea. Go to a Twelve Step meeting and you'll meet a mix of people, some who are new to recovery, others who are coming back from a relapse after varying periods of sobriety, always a core group of people with many years of continuous sobriety. They are living proof that consistently attending meetings and working a Twelve Step program one day at a time is probably the best way to have days turn to months and months to years, as the rewards of sober living accumulate.

Still, anything can trigger us to step on the trap. As we noted in our formula above, sometimes we relapse because we're obsessed with the idea that "it'll be different this time," that we'll control how much we use and when, because we've learned from the mistakes of our past. As one addict put it, "Nobody had to convince me that using drugs was a bad idea. My problem was thinking I had a better idea [of] how to use them."

Another factor is our tendency to use chemicals to medicate our emotions. We may not even be conscious of doing it. Remember, we used substances to alter how we experienced life's highs and lows. We used them to mitigate the negative feelings about ourselves and the people around us whose expectations we weren't meeting. You could say that we used them to medicate the pain of our shortcomings, real and perceived, and to artificially boost our egos. When we stop using, we are likely to experience our emotions like never before. Much of regaining this ability to feel our feelings again is exciting and rewarding, but it can also be difficult and may feel unfair. We may find ourselves musing, "I thought quitting drugs was supposed to make me feel better." If we aren't careful, if we don't stay focused on recovery as a process with both hardships and rewards, if we allow the craving of the mind and the thirst of the spirit to pull us off course, we will find ourselves walking not only into a steel trap but into a minefield.

We've talked about how this can be true even after decades of sobriety. I know of a man who achieved recovery, became an addiction counselor, and became a legend among his peers. His family noticed first that he had stopped taking care of himself and was pouring all his energy into his professional role and feeding off the self-esteem that his success gave him. After thirty years, he retired and suddenly found himself void of the professional identity he had relished and the sense of purpose that had driven him to stay sober. The "phenomenon of craving" returned. He took a drink. That inevitably led to more drinks. One day he passed out in the bathroom at his home, struck his head on the toilet, and died. The official cause of death: fractured skull. The real cause of death: his chronic illness, alcoholism. His case is proof that this is a progressive disease and that no matter how long we're abstinent, if we relapse, the illness has continued to progress and we may likely be worse off than when we first quit.

TEACHABLE MOMENTS

German philosopher Friedrich Nietzsche said, "What doesn't kill us makes us stronger." So it can be with relapse. The pain, embarrassment, and shame of relapse usually leaves us down and out and despairing once again, asking ourselves, "Now what?" But our recovery experience can be different this time—if we can keep our original commitment to get and stay sober in perspective with what's gone awry. A relapse can become a teachable moment if we take the time to connect the dots. Connect them and eventually this is the picture that emerges:

The choice to take the first drink or hit is yours alone.

Nobody made you do it. Although you might not yet know exactly why you did it, you can recount the events as they unfolded, from the moment the idea popped into your head to the split second before you put into your body the substance that you knew would disrupt your life as the craving for more took over. You can then make a commitment to avoid the people, places, and things that triggered the thought that you could use again without negative consequences. This isn't about blame or finding fault. It is, however, about accountability. This is your chance to own your addiction and to take the necessary steps to get back on the path to recovery.

There was probably plenty of opportunity to prevent your relapse right up until the moment you did it.

If only you had honestly shared your thoughts and feelings with somebody in a position to help you—a family member, a recovery coach or sponsor, your counselor, a friend or "fellow traveler" in your circle of recovery, anyone—before the dealer or bartender handed you your drug of choice. Stealth and secrets are a driving force of addiction and, therefore, of relapse. We addicts are notorious for keeping quiet and looking good on the outside even as our brains scream for a hit or a drink and we are falling apart inside. Nobody I know has ever relapsed if he first told the right person what he was about to do. There is nothing wrong with wanting to get high again. Keeping it to yourself, however, can be a deadly problem.

Addiction is an inconvenient illness.

It's easy to resent having to take time out to recover from it. This is especially true after the acute crisis has passed, when you feel better, but you've only just started to put back together what was fractured. It's also easy for the efforts required to stay substance-free to slip further and further down your "to do" list, with kids to raise, a demanding job, school, marriage counseling, summer vacation, a sick parent to care for, the holidays, mowing the lawn, and everything else that life demands and also give us as rewards. You may have altogether stopped making any special efforts in working a recovery program. Look at your calendar in the days and weeks before you tripped up. Take an inventory of what you did the past couple of months. Where were your recovery-related activities? Did you do those things that you'd been told would keep your sobriety firm—for example, practicing daily meditation, attending recovery meetings, reading recovery literature, pitching in to help others?

When we're not actively taking responsibility for our recovery, we're coasting.

"We coast in only one direction, downward," George Weller, an addiction counselor, told me more than once. Even before we get to the point that we take the drink or drug again, we've already lapsed into the same pattern of behaviors that are all about our addictive personality, which is characterized by dishonesty, selfishness, and resentment. When we start acting like the addict of old, we're bound to start using like one. We lose pace in keeping ahead of our illness. It snaps at our heels. Suddenly it catches and then overtakes us. We're high again.

A lot of people relapse because they don't pay attention to what else is happening in their bodies.

Emotional pain and mental illness can blindside even the most committed alcoholic and addict in recovery. If you don't get the professional help you need and then follow the counselor's treatment plan, including taking appropriate nonaddictive medications, it won't be long before you're askew. Once out of balance, you'll lose perspective and know those feelings again that you were medicating with alcohol and other drugs in the first place. This is also true if you suffer from physical ailments, such as high blood pressure, an overactive thyroid, or premenstrual syndrome (PMS), that require medications. When we feel lousy mentally or physically, we're vulnerable. Take care of yourself—body, mind, and spirit.

A drug is a drug is a drug—that's all that matters to you.

If your drug of choice isn't prescription painkillers and your doctor wants to prescribe them for pain, you will be very tempted to not tell him or her that you're an addict. Maybe you don't think you have to, because it's only medicine, and medicine prescribed by a doctor is good for you, right? Why suffer? Suddenly you're enraptured with a new lover, and, if you're not abusing the new drugs, you'll be in danger of being reminded of the "good old days" and will be right back where you started, or worse, with your drug of choice, or worse. It's also common for addicts to take up gambling, pornography, and other compulsive behaviors that trigger the same brain chemicals that some drugs do. Then they find themselves in the throes of addiction again, the only difference being the name of the drug. The key is to remember that abstinence doesn't just apply to your drug of choice but to all mood-altering chemicals and compulsive behaviors.

If you've made these connections, perhaps now you understand how your relapse unfolded. If you've so far avoided stepping into the trap, you make these connections and your prospects to stay on the sober and drug-free path improve, especially as the years go by. Most important, stay teachable. Relapse doesn't mean starting over. It means starting again by starting differently, this time with more self-knowledge and a renewed commitment to recovery.

In my recovery journey, what I've learned through the years to keep me sober has as much to do with coming to terms with what I did wrong or realizing what I can do better as it does with what I've done right. Relapse is never a goal. But if it happens, then make it your goal to take from relapse what is required to avoid it the next time.

RELAPSE AND THE FAMILY

The first time addiction intrudes on a family and everyone finally picks up and puts back together the pieces, there's the hope and belief it won't happen again.

And when an addict relapses, usually the family members do, too, right back into the behaviors, thoughts, feelings, and responses that caught them up in the whirlwind of addiction the first time.

To illustrate, here is one mother's story:

> When my husband and I attended the family program, the counselor spoke about relapse. She warned us that relapse is very common but doesn't indicate failure. Inside my head, though, I was saying, "Not my son. Now that he has been sober for six weeks, I feel certain that he is healing and will never use or drink again. After all, he is a wonderful person who has shown many times all his life that he is disciplined, smart, and has a solid spiritual foundation. And furthermore, he wants very badly to be well again and get back to his good life."

For this mother's son, all of this was true. Early in his recovery he was confident. His faith was restored. He had a decent head on his shoulders and a career to get back to soon. His family stood by him and with him. Only thirty, his body quickly healed, his mind refocused. He felt restored. Except that he failed in a fundamental understanding that treatment is the beginning of a lifelong process. That addiction in remission is still addiction lurking. Yes, he had heard others talk of the pitfalls of relapse. But he was supremely confident, like his mother. Too confident, it turns out. His mother tells us what happened next:

Little did I know that he would experience the misery of relapse several times. Within a very short time, he was in treatment again, the second time. All the family was shaken to our bones as we began to realize that his recovery would be full of ups and downs and dangers and crashes. How many times could we hold up to this frightening reality?

I began to absorb the faces of every homeless man I met on the street or stepped around in the subway. Could my handsome, clean-cut, well-educated son ever become homeless and lost? Would we lose all contact with him as he fell into the terrible pit of long-term despair? I had nightmares of finding him in a morgue somewhere.

Sleepless nights and numbing days at work led me to increase the number of Twelve Step meetings I attended and to get private counseling sessions. Faced with the possibilities of extended worry and struggle, I had to learn to let go of the idea that I could somehow save him. I realized that I must face my own issues and realities.

Finally one night I dreamed that I was standing next to his open casket. I studied his familiar face and remembered it as a baby, a toddler, a Boy Scout, a teenager, a caring adult. And then I closed the lid of that casket. When I awoke, I had a feeling of peace.

It was not the separation from the connection of mother and son. I continued to love him and to stand behind him in appropriate ways. But I had to learn the meaning of *appropriate.*

When I introduce myself in a Twelve Step meeting, I say, "I'm Judith, and I'm a 'fixer.'" It's true that in my job as a television producer and CEO I am required to make things happen, to correct mistakes, to create. And in my personal life, I love to decorate my home, care for the garden, cook, give parties. I am a good fixer. I love to fix. But I have needed to learn—and am still learning—where to draw the line, where to stop, how not to try to fix people.

But family members have relapses too. Sometimes I need renewal through some new readings and sessions, extra meetings, even occasionally a brief retreat. And, in my tradition, more attention to meditation and prayer.

That storyteller is Judith Moyers, my mother. And although she has always been my steadfast pillar of support, my relapses through the years drained even her seemingly limitless reserve of hope to the point of exhaustion. Quite simply, she ran out of patience and energy at the same time I ran out of options.

Or in the words of Marcy S., whose son Scott relapsed, "I am trying very hard to step back this time and let him do it on his own, but I'm his mother, and mothers are supposed to be there for their children all the time. This is the hardest thing in the world."

It is never easy for a family to stick to the principles of the "three C's" that they're told about over and over again in the course of their loved one's travails. Objectively, on paper, the points make perfect sense: "I didn't *cause*, can't *cure*, and can't *control* what's happening to the addict." But embracing this approach is like telling somebody who's unemployed not to dream about winning the lottery. That's fine for everybody else. But we think, "You're talking about the person I love, and I don't want that person to suffer, or my worst fear, to die."

What do you do, though, when each relapse is like a ruptured oil well, spilling so much pollution that it's hard to know how or where to start the cleanup, even as the damage continues to spread?

I think it's similar to the approach described in my "Four Steps to Sanity" column in chapter 3, how the successful, loving father deals with his daughter who chooses to continue drinking:

- Love the person even if you hate what relapse has done to them, and keep reminding them of this love-hate dynamic.
- Forgive the addict while at the same time offering to help them get help—but balance it with clear, stout boundaries that affirm your expectations and need to protect your own wellness.
- Never give up hope. Without it there won't be another opportunity to take action if and when the addict is finally ready for help.

- Don't endure this process all by yourself, any more than you want the addict to go it alone, either.

Do this as the veteran you now are, for by this point you'll have intimate knowledge of addiction, especially if you've watched the person you love relapse repeatedly. The relapses still make you angry, hurt, frustrated, and scared. That's natural. You have a right to feel this way. But eventually, you'll face the hard reality that when you can't do anything else, you need to take care of yourself. You'll still be tempted to fall back on popular bromides, such as "Families should do anything for the people they love, even at the cost of our own well-being." No more, though. The only real power you have is to empower yourself. This isn't to suggest you simply sit idly by. You still can keep the lines of communication open and be there should the addict decide to take responsibility for her own recovery.

And remember that you aren't the only one going through this. Many families who have been put through the ringer by relapse find support in Al-Anon and Alateen. You can join them in saying that you're "in recovery" even when the addict isn't. Often what is shared in these meetings is the frustration regarding the inability to "let go" and the recurring, irrational desire to grab on to the addict once more in the belief that, this time, you can help them see the light. The wisdom in Al-Anon doesn't come out of a textbook. It is birthed and nurtured and shared among people who understand their limitations and are learning that they deserve to live full lives, even if the addicts they love are destroying theirs. Al-Anon reminds us that we don't have to do it alone.

Not long after Marcy S. wrote me pleading "Help, my son is dying" she scraped together a few thousand dollars and sent Scott to Minnesota, where he got help. "I was looking for the strength to stop drinking and I found it," he told me. "I don't want to go back to that way of life where alcohol controls all of me."

For some time Scott did well. But then he took a few drinks, stopped again, drank some more, and soon couldn't pull out of his spiral. In the middle of the night he called me in despair, drunk. "I can't do this anymore. I'm dying." But he kept drinking.

Marcy reached out to me again, not sure what to do, even though she was already doing it.

"He's locked himself in his apartment and told his roommate he wants to die. For my own sanity I've stayed completely away from him for over a month now, no communication at all except he said 'Happy birthday' a few weeks ago, and I said 'Thank you.' I have never in his life not seen or talked to him for this long. My question is, do you think I am doing the right thing? Time and time again I've tried to help him . . . now he does not have money to pay his rent, so he will be out on the street next week. Do you think I should let him fall all the way down? It is very hard for me but I have survived the month. I'm just asking because I am so afraid he will try to do himself in once his roommate leaves. He's totally alone and out on the street. I need to know I am doing the right thing, I guess."

A few days later she sent me this update.

"I could not leave my son alone any longer—mother's intuition—and when I got to his apartment he was passed out, semi-comatose . . . he was taken to the hospital with a

.45 [blood alcohol content]. The doctors say he would have died within a few more hours if I hadn't gone there. It is so hard to stick to a boundary. I know it is important to take care of myself. I know I can't make him stop drinking or get help. But this time I am glad I didn't turn my back on him. I'm doing what I can for him and for me."

Then a few days later, this:

"He is out of the hospital and getting his strength back. I did what I know I shouldn't and let him come back home for as long as I am still here. I pray it will work out for a while . . . so much is coming at him now since he's lost his job: mammoth hospital bills and all the other consequences. I've told him he can stay only a few weeks because I have decided to put my house up for sale . . . financially I just can't make it anymore. But anyway, he has been helping me to get things done with the house. I begged him to go to Minnesota for help while he was in the hospital, but I know this is his choice so there is not much I can do. I am starting to realize that I have no control: whatever will be, will be. So hard! So hard! All I can do is pray that he changes his mind. I can't change it for him. The only think I can change is my thinking! I'm doing my best taking care of myself now."

Marcy's "Now what?" is the dilemma of everyone who loves an addict or an alcoholic who won't get help or can't stop using. She did her part for her son. The result—*I am starting to realize that I have no control: whatever will be, will be*—won't solve her son's problem. But for now, it answers hers.

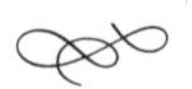

EPILOGUE

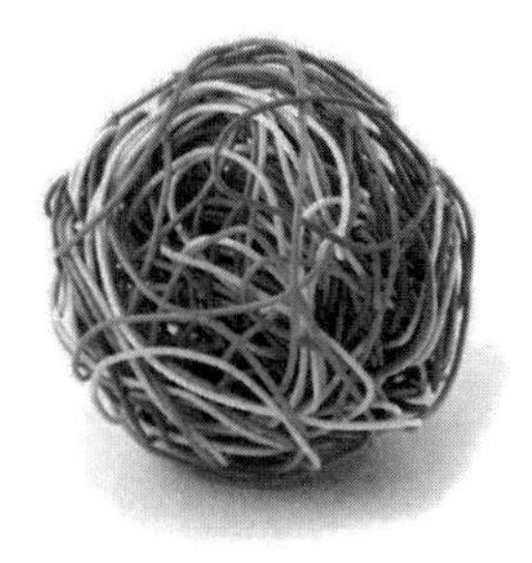

"Pass It On"

There's an AA slogan, "Pass it on," that sums up Step Twelve's challenge to "carry this message to alcoholics, and to practice these principles in all our affairs." For me that has meant not only going to meetings, doing my public speaking, and writing books like this. It has also meant trying to pass on what I've learned and who I've become in recovery to the next generation, starting with my own children.

Of all the online columns I've written, "Token of Gratitude," which appeared in October 2009, elicited the largest number of responses. I'd like to share it with you here.

For his seventeenth birthday, I gave my oldest son a gift certificate to fill up his truck with gasoline a couple of times. He drives an old Chevy Tahoe, so the card won't take him very far. But with some cash he got from his grandparents and his job mowing a neighbor's lawn, he's got a reserve to keep him rolling along for a couple of months.

What I hope he'll get more mileage out of is my other small present to him, a metal token with Roman numeral XVII stamped on one side and the Serenity Prayer on the other. It's the kind of medallion that's typically given to alcoholics and addicts to mark their journey in recovery. Such tokens include amounts as small as twenty-four hours to as long as multiple decades.

My son isn't an alcoholic. In fact, he says he's never taken a drink or used a drug, and I believe him. But a few days before his birthday, I realized that by my seventeenth birthday in 1976, I had started to experiment with marijuana and beer, sparking a chain reaction to full-blown addiction that I did not overcome until I was thirty-five years old. I've been clean and sober since 1994. My oldest has been the same since 1992, when he was born.

So I gave him the medallion to recognize my appreciation that he has, at least so far, stayed away from those substances. The medallion was in a hand-carved wooden box with this note to him:

Dear Son:

When I was your age, I had already started the slow slide into trouble caused by my decision to experiment with alcohol and other drugs. On your seventeenth birthday, this medallion honors the admirable choice you have made to live these years up to now without them. I hope and pray you'll add more tokens to this special keepsake box in the years ahead. I am so proud of you.

Love,
Dad

On the Sunday after his birthday, my son and his other brother (who at fifteen also has been "clean" as long as I have) and I watched the Minnesota Vikings battle the Pittsburgh Steelers on television. During those three hours of football, about a dozen commercials pitched various brands of beer. Those ads were mostly funny, cleverly done, and engaging, even to the three of us. So I am no fool. From Madison Avenue advertising to websites for online pharmacies selling Viagra to Vicoden, access is easy and temptation is ubiquitous, especially for teenagers, mine included.

All I can do is lead by example. I stay sober in front of my kids by sharing with them what it was like for me at their ages, what happened, and why I must continue to take care of myself all these years later. I encourage them to learn from their father, and I remind them that if they choose to use mood- and mind-altering substances, they may not be able to choose the outcome. But I also emphasize that if they develop a problem, it is okay to ask me for help.

In the meantime, I'll keep giving them medallions. Whether just for today or for longer, they need to know that I value their efforts to make the right choices in their journeys through these tricky teenage years and beyond.

"Would you take me to one of those meetings you go to for recovery?" my son asked me one day.

And that's when it hit me, both in my own life and at the moment I was finishing this book. The real-life experiences that became our stories that became the chapters are always punctuated by "Now what?" mileposts when the roiling confusion of alcohol or other drugs blocks a clear escape route from our predicament, whether we are the addict in trouble or we love the addict who needs help. So often are we desperate for an answer, lonely, scared, and unsure where to turn—until we suddenly discover the problem isn't ours to solve all by ourselves.

Because addiction is a disease of isolation, the antidote is togetherness, other people, community—moving from "I" to "we." Chris Edrington, founder of St. Paul Sober Living, a network of residential homes for addicts and alcoholics integrated into the larger neighborhoods in the Twin Cities and Coloraro, says this:

> When we're using and when we're behaving in the culture around using, we're keeping ourselves out of the relationships that we need to be in, like with

> family and with people who are having success and having things work out in their lives. And it's a real difficult perception to have in early sobriety, it's really difficult to see the big picture. We're very self-focused in the early days. That's why it's important to surround yourself with people who are positive about recovery. Live with them. Work with them. Hang out with them. Get involved as much as you can, and be part of the core. Stay in the middle of the herd is the analogy, so you don't get picked off. And inside of that process, all kinds of stuff starts working out.

Whether you're an alcoholic or addict or someone asking "Now what?" I hope that if you've gotten nothing else from this book, you've learned that you don't have to face your challenges alone. We are surrounded by generations of addicts, their families, and friends who know exactly where we've been and who have lived the answers to "Now what?" Remember: Their stories are your story too. Don't forget to pass it on.

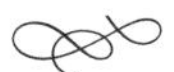

APPENDIX A

RESOURCES FOR GETTING HELP

For Alcoholics and Addicts

Alcoholics Anonymous World Services, www.aa.org

Narcotics Anonymous World Services, www.na.org

Substance Abuse and Mental Health Services Administration (SAMHSA) treatment finder, www.samhsa.gov/treatment

Hazelden Foundation, www.hazelden.org / 24-hour helpline: 800-257-7810

Alcoholics Anonymous, fourth edition. New York: Alcoholics Anonymous World Services, Inc., 2001

Narcotics Anonymous, sixth edition. Van Nuys, CA: Narcotics Anonymous World Services, Inc., 2008

Getting Started in AA, by Hamilton B. Center City, MN: Hazelden, 1995

Finding a Home Group, by James G. Center City, MN: Hazelden, 2011

Undrunk: A Skeptic's Guide to AA, by A. J. Adams. Center City, MN: Hazelden, 2009

Twenty-Four Hours a Day. Center City, MN: Hazelden, 1975

Each Day a New Beginning: Daily Meditations for Women, by Karen Casey. Center City, MN: Hazelden, 1982

A Woman's Way through the Twelve Steps, by Stephanie Covington. Center City, MN: Hazelden, 1994

For Families

Addict in the Family: Stories of Loss, Hope, and Recovery, by Beverly Conyers. Center City, MN: Hazelden, 2003

Al-Anon Family Groups, www. Al-anon.alateen.org

Nar-Anon Family Groups, www.nar-anon.org

Co-Dependents Anonymous World Fellowship (CoDA), www.coda.org

Everything Changes: Help for Families of Newly Recovering Addicts, by Beverly Conyers. Center City, MN: Hazelden, 2009

How Al-Anon Works: for Families and Friends of Alcoholics. Virginia Beach, VA: Al-Anon Family Group Headquarters, Inc., 1995

Detachment and Enabling, by Rebecca D. Chaitin and Judith M. Knowlton. Center City, MN: Hazelden, 1985

Codependent No More: How to Stop Controlling Others and Start Caring for Yourself, by Melody Beattie. Center City, MN: Hazelden, 1986

It Will Never Happen to Me: Growing Up with Addiction as Youngsters, Adolescents, Adults, by Claudia Black, PhD. Center City, MN: Hazelden, 2002

Language of Letting Go, by Melody Beattie. Center City, MN: Hazelden, 1990

Love First: A Family's Guide to Intervention, second edition, by Jeff Jay and Debra Jay. Center City, MN: Hazelden, 2008

APPENDIX B

THE DRUG ABUSE SCREENING TEST: DAST-20

This basic test consists of twenty questions. Answering "yes" to six or more of the questions (except for questions 4 and 5, to which you would count a "no" answer) indicates a likely diagnosis of substance abuse or dependence.

1. Have you used drugs other than those required for medical reasons? ___Yes ___No
2. Have you abused prescription drugs? ___Yes ___No
3. Do you abuse more than one drug at a time? ___Yes ___No
4. Can you get through the week without using drugs? ___Yes ___No
5. Are you always able to stop using drugs when you want to? ___Yes ___No
6. Have you had "blackouts" or "flashbacks" as a result of drug use? ___Yes ___No
7. Do you ever feel bad or guilty about your drug use? ___Yes ___No
8. Does your spouse (or parents) ever complain about your involvement with drugs? ___Yes ___No
9. Has drug abuse created problems between you and your spouse or your parents? ___Yes ___No

10. Have you lost friends because of your use of drugs? ___Yes ___No

11. Have you neglected your family because of your use of drugs? ___Yes ___No

12. Have you been in trouble at work because of your use of drugs? ___Yes ___No

13. Have you lost a job because of drug abuse? ___Yes ___No

14. Have you gotten into fights when under the influence of drugs? ___Yes ___No

15. Have you engaged in illegal activities in order to obtain drugs? ___Yes ___No

16. Have you been arrested for possession of illegal drugs? ___Yes ___No

17. Have you ever experienced withdrawal symptoms (felt sick) when you stopped taking a drug? ___Yes ___No

18. Have you had medical problems as a result of your drug use (e.g., memory loss, hepatitis, convulsions, bleeding, etc.)? ___Yes ___No

19. Have you gone to anyone for help for a drug problem? ___Yes ___No

20. Have you been involved in a treatment program especially related to drug use? ___Yes ___No

APPENDIX C

YOUR PLAN FOR THE FIRST FIVE DAYS SOBER AND DRUG-FREE

Adapted from William Moyers's *A New Day, A New Life*
(Center City, MN: Hazelden, 2009).
Used with permission.

DAY ONE: CREATE A SAFE SPACE

Your first recovery action step is to "trash your stash"—to clear your living environment of every last bit of alcohol or other drugs. Get rid of any materials (posters, music, shot glasses, phone numbers of using friends) that remind you of drinking or using. Don't do this alone. Ask your spouse, domestic partner, sober friend, or supportive family member for help.

You might be tempted to save part of your stash. Realize that this thinking will set you up for certain failure. Get rid of *all* your stash, and trust that you can let go of the need to control your life by using substances.

Write down the name of a sober person you can trust and schedule a time to meet to get rid of your stash within the next twenty-four hours. It's hard, but you can do it.

DAY TWO: FIND A LOCAL TWELVE STEP MEETING

Alcoholics Anonymous (AA) or Narcotics Anonymous (NA) Twelve Step meetings offer a fellowship where recovering people share their experience, strength, and hope. Going to AA meetings is especially important during the first year of recovery. You, like many others, may have felt isolated and lonely, as though you "didn't belong." Using alcohol or other drugs probably made that alienation even worse. What is the best cure for alienation and isolation? Friendship. When you make a connection with others in AA, loneliness will decrease. If you have a problem, question, or experience you don't understand, you can turn to a fellow AA member for help.

Use the Internet or your local phone book to find a Twelve Step meeting in your area. Make a commitment to go to a meeting during the next twenty-four hours, and plan to go at least once a week. Write down the address of the meeting and list the day and time you will attend.

Read the Big Book, *Alcoholics Anonymous,* page 58–71 (4th ed.), "How It Works." Describe any fears or doubts you have about how the Twelve Step program can help you. Share these doubts in a Twelve Step meeting you attend this week.

DAY THREE: FIND A SPONSOR

Twelve Step recovery is based on the idea that healing begins when you become willing to share your story with another person. In early recovery the first person you share with is called a sponsor. When you find a sponsor, you will have a special person who can listen to your story with attentive ears and an understanding heart.

Your sponsor will support, challenge, and help you in times of crisis and guide you through your Twelve Step work. It is not a sponsor's duty to keep you sober or take the place of a trained counselor; it is your sponsor's job to hold you accountable and assist you in building a healthy lifestyle.

When you attend your first Twelve Step meeting, make sure you don't leave without finding a temporary sponsor who is your same gender. A few people in your meeting will likely offer to be your temporary sponsor, but make sure you ask for help if you need it.

Your temporary sponsor will help guide you through the first few weeks or months of recovery. After you get to know people in your meeting better, you may always choose a different sponsor who fits your needs more perfectly. But right now make sure you identify someone who will be your sponsor. Program his or her phone number into your cell phone or keep it in your wallet.

DAY FOUR: UNDERSTAND THE BRAIN SCIENCE OF ADDICTION

Research has shown that addiction is not a matter of an individual's strength, moral character, willpower, or weakness. It has to do with brain chemistry and the way your brain is "wired." When you used drugs or alcohol, your bloodstream quickly carried powerful, feel-good chemicals called neurotransmitters to your brain, causing you to feel high. This feeling was so pleasurable that you wanted to repeat it again and again.

Eventually your body got used to the drug and needed more to feel high. Eventually your brain stopped producing feel-good neurotransmitters on its own. Ordinary things like good food, a sunny day, or making a friend laugh no longer made you happy. Your body had become a hostage to the drug and you could not feel happy—or even normal—without it.

Your body was chemically out of balance, and your need to use was more powerful than your best intentions to quit. Because you couldn't quit, your drug use became progressively worse.

Can you relate to this description of how addiction progresses? Take a few minutes to reflect on your first use of alcohol or other drugs. How did your drug use progress? When did you notice that you needed the drug just to feel "normal"?

DAY FIVE: PLAN YOUR DAY

In early recovery you cannot be around any mood-altering substances. To stay safe, you will need to plan your day to avoid being around *all* people and places that could cause you to use alcohol or other drugs. It's extremely important for you to stay away from bars or other places that remind you of using.

Don't fool yourself into thinking you can drink or use like your nonaddicted buddies, because you can't. Your brain is wired differently. Walking into a bar or meeting your using friends at a park is a "slippery slope" that will lead right back to drug use. Nonaddicts can have one drink and go home, but for addicts, one drink can easily turn into ten.

Think about the "slippery places" where you previously used alcohol or other drugs. Did you use when you were home alone? With friends? First thing after waking up in the morning? At concerts? Before or during a date? After payday?

List these slippery places and make a commitment to avoid them at all costs. Instead of going to a bar or over to a using friend's house, write out a plan to go to a Twelve Step meeting, connect with a sober friend, or go to a coffee shop or a bookstore.

APPENDIX D

WRITING AN INTERVENTION LETTER

Reprinted from Jeff and Debra Jay's *Love First,* 2nd edition
(Center City, MN: Hazelden, 2008).
Used with permission.

Begin your letter with a salutation, such as *Dear Dad* or *Dear Kathy.* End your letter by referring to your relationship, such as *Your best friend, Kay.* Stating your relationship is powerful. It may seem silly since you and the alcoholic are sitting in the same room, but it isn't. These words have a deep emotional impact.

End your letter by directly asking the alcoholic to accept help. Make it clear that you are asking him to take immediate action by including words like *today* or *now.* The entire purpose of writing your letter is ultimately to ask one question, "Will you accept the help we're offering you today?" Everyone's letter should end with a similar question.

As you write, stay in first person. Don't speak for the group, only for yourself. Instead of writing *we all love you,* write *I love you.* By using *we* instead of *I,* you dilute the emotional force of your message. Only use *we* when you specifically want to refer to the intervention group, such as in your final question, "Will you accept the help we are offering you today?"

We have created guidelines to follow when writing your intervention letter. By using this seven-point format, composing your letter will be simpler.

1. Introduction

Write a brief opening statement of love that specifically states the nature of your relationship. ("Jack, I have been very lucky to have you as my best friend for more than twenty years. Not many people in this world have the good fortune to have a friend like you.")

2. Love

This is the longest part of the letter. Do not bring up problems related to addiction in this part of the letter. Instead, give specific reasons why you love and care about the person, remembering times when you were proud of her, when she was there for you, fun times you experienced together, examples of her best character traits. This part of the letter must be sincere, avoiding empty flattery. If the addict's behavior has been difficult for a long time, remember back to better days. ("Carrie, I can remember back like it was yesterday to the day I asked you to marry me. You were so beautiful as we walked through the snow. When I looked at you, I thought my heart would burst. I'd never before known a girl like you. . . .")

3. Reframing

Shift from the love section to a discussion of the problem by stating your understanding of addiction as a genetic disease. Differentiate addiction from character and willpower issues. Talk about the need for professional treatment. If other people in your family have suffered from alcoholism, mention that it runs in the family. ("Michael, problems with alcohol dependence affects one out of eight people who drink, because it is a genetic, inherited disease. You didn't choose this any more than Dad chose diabetes. Alcoholism runs in our family. Our great-grandfather was an alcoholic, and Aunt Kate became addicted to prescription drugs. It requires professional treatment just like any other disease.")

4. Facts

Provide specific, firsthand examples of problems caused by alcohol or other drugs. Don't use judgmental or angry language. Don't try to tell the addict what he or she was thinking. Instead, describe what you saw and how you felt. Let the facts speak for themselves. Be brief. One to three examples is sufficient, and don't dredge up ancient history unless there is a very good reason to do so. ("Patti, alcohol is making decisions in your life I know you would never make for yourself. Last week you drove the kids to soccer practice after you'd been drinking. You're a great mom, and I don't believe you'd ever do that if there weren't a problem with alcohol. The kids have told me that sometimes you smell of beer when you pick them up from school. Two nights ago, I heard you slurring your words when you put them to bed. I see alcohol hurting you, and it's hurting them. And I hurt, too.")

5. Commitment

Make a personal commitment to stand by the alcoholic and help him or her in any way that is possible and appropriate. ("I have learned that this is a family disease. It requires that we all participate in the recovery process. I am pledging to do my part. I will attend the family program and Al-Anon. Together, we will heal and we will grow. It'll be a wonderful journey as a family.")

6. Ask

This is a direct request that the alcoholic immediately accept the treatment program being offered. One team member can add a few lines in their letter about the treatment center you've selected. If the treatment center provides special programs or amenities that will be of interest to your loved one, mention them. ("Josh, we have taken the time to find the best program for you. It's a great facility in the mountains with an outward-bound wilderness experience. It's a special program for people in your age range—young men in their teens and early twenties. We think you'll really like it. Will you accept the help we're offering you today?")

7. Affirmation

End on a positive note, painting a positive picture of the future. Give your loved one a reason to want to get sober. Speak of ways the addict is important to you and others. Give him a sense of purpose. Express faith in his ability to follow through and succeed. ("Dad, I need you in my life. You are my rock. I'm graduating from college next year, and Sean and I have been talking about getting married. I need you healthy to walk me down the aisle. I want you to be the best grandfather for my children. It's you I want to lean on in the tough times and celebrate with in the good times. I love you, Dad. I want you back.")

Give yourself plenty of time to write your letter. Some people write their letter one day and revise it the next. Write from the heart. During the intervention training, share letters with each other. Read them aloud during the rehearsal. Make necessary edits. Remove any language that could make the alcoholic or addict angry or defensive. Rewrite your letters to incorporate changes so they are neat and easy to read. Don't leave scribbles or notes in the margins. Always use loving, nonjudgmental honesty when talking about the problem. Throw your heart into the love section of the letter.

When your loved one goes into treatment, deliver all letters to the treatment staff. If he or she refuses treatment, have the interventionist, chairperson, or another appropriate team member deliver the letters to your addicted loved one at the earliest possible time. Team members should keep a copy of the letter they've written for themselves.

APPENDIX E

The Twelve Steps of Alcoholics Anonymous

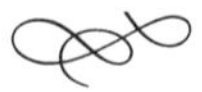

1. We admitted we were powerless over alcohol—that our lives had become unmanageable.
2. Came to believe that a Power greater than ourselves could restore us to sanity.
3. Made a decision to turn our will and our lives over to the care of God *as we understood Him.*
4. Made a searching and fearless moral inventory of ourselves.
5. Admitted to God, to ourselves, and to another human being the exact nature of our wrongs.
6. Were entirely ready to have God remove all these defects of character.
7. Humbly asked Him to remove our shortcomings.
8. Made a list of all persons we had harmed, and became willing to make amends to them all.
9. Made direct amends to such people wherever possible, except when to do so would injure them or others.
10. Continued to take personal inventory and when we were wrong promptly admitted it.
11. Sought through prayer and meditation to improve our conscious contact with God *as we understood Him,* praying only for knowledge of His will for us and the power to carry that out.
12. Having had a spiritual awakening as the result of these Steps, we tried to carry this message to alcoholics, and to practice these principles in all our affairs.

Reprinted from *Alcoholics Anonymous,* 4th ed.
(New York: Alcoholics Anonymous World Services, 2001), 59–60.

APPENDIX F

THE TWELVE STEPS OF NARCOTICS ANONYMOUS

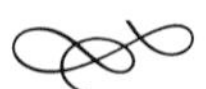

1. We admitted that we were powerless over our addiction, that our lives had become unmanageable.
2. We came to believe that a Power greater than ourselves could restore us to sanity.
3. We made a decision to turn our will and our lives over to the care of God as we understood Him.
4. We made a searching and fearless moral inventory of ourselves.
5. We admitted to God, to ourselves, and to another human being the exact nature of our wrongs.
6. We were entirely ready to have God remove all these defects of character.
7. We humbly asked Him to remove our shortcomings.
8. We made a list of all persons we had harmed, and became willing to make amends to them all.
9. We made direct amends to such people wherever possible, except when to do so would injure them or others.
10. We continued to take personal inventory and when we were wrong promptly admitted it.
11. We sought through prayer and meditation to improve our conscious contact with God as we understood Him, praying only for knowledge of His will for us and the power to carry that out.
12. Having had a spiritual awakening as a result of these steps, we tried to carry this message to addicts, and to practice these principles in all our affairs.

Reprinted from *Narcotics Anonymous,* 6th ed.
(Chatsworth, CA: Narcotics Anonymous World Services, 2008), 17.